112 Sleep Improving Juice and Meal Recipes:

Eating Right So You Can Sleep Better at Night without Having to Take Pills

By

Joe Correa CSN

COPYRIGHT

This publication is designed to provide accurate and authoritative information in regard to the subject matter covered. It is sold with the understanding that neither the author nor the publisher is engaged in rendering medical advice. If medical advice or assistance is needed, consult with a doctor. This book is considered a guide and should not be used in any way detrimental to your health. Consult with a physician before starting this nutritional plan to make sure it's right for you.

ACKNOWLEDGEMENTS

This book is dedicated to my friends and family that have had mild or serious illnesses so that you may find a solution and make the necessary changes in your life.

112 Sleep Improving Juice and Meal Recipes:

Eating Right So You Can Sleep Better at Night without Having to Take Pills

By

Joe Correa CSN

CONTENTS

ABOUT THE AUTHOR

After years of Research, I honestly believe in the positive effects that proper nutrition can have over the body and mind. My knowledge and experience has helped me live healthier throughout the years and which I have shared with family and friends. The more you know about eating and drinking healthier, the sooner you will want to change your life and eating habits.

Nutrition is a key part in the process of being healthy and living longer so get started today. The first step is the most important and the most significant.

INTRODUCTION

112 Sleep Improving Juice and Meal Recipes: Eating Right So You Can Sleep Better at Night without Having to Take Pills

By Joe Correa CSN

A lot of different factors can affect a good night sleep and create sleep disorders and other sleep-related problems. The most common problems include snoring, insomnia, sleep deprivation, and restless legs syndrome. Having some of these symptoms can have serious effects on your life and you might find yourself feeling depressed and irritable, struggling to remember information, and craving unhealthy foods.

Sleep disorders are linked to weight gain and obesity. Individuals who tend to sleep less have a bigger appetite and eat more calories that usually come from unhealthy and highly-processed foods. Furthermore, lack of sleep affects the hormones and causes poor appetite regulation by reducing the levels of leptin, the hormone that suppresses appetite. Poor sleepers, on the other hand, are at far greater risk of heart disease. When combined together, these two side effects can create a serious and life-threatening condition.

The bottom line is that 7-8 hours of quality sleep per night is crucial for overall health and well-being. The good news is that there is a lot you can do about it. There are certain foods that are proven to help or affect your sleep.

About 60% of people in the world sleep between six and eight hours a day, 36% sleep more than eight hours a day, while less than 4% sleep less than six hours. Both, men and women have the same need for sleep.

These sleep improving juice and meal recipes will help you get more rest at night by providing your body with soothing and relaxing foods. Try them all and see which ones help you sleep and stay asleep.

112 SLEEP IMPROVING JUICE AND MEAL RECIPES: EATING RIGHT SO YOU CAN SLEEP BETTER AT NIGHT WITHOUT HAVING TO TAKE PILLS

MEALS

1.   Warm Quinoa with Bananas and Chia Seeds

Ingredients:

- 2 tsp of chia seeds, soaked

- ½ cup of almond milk

- 1.5oz quinoa

- ½ cup of water

- 1 small banana, peeled and sliced

- 2 tbsp of blueberries

- 1 tbsp of honey

- 1 tbsp of almonds, roughly chopped

Preparation:

Combine the water and almond milk in a medium sized

saucepan. Bring it to a boil and add quinoa. Reduce the heat and cook for about 20 minutes, or until all the water evaporates.

Meanwhile, mash ½ banana with a fork. Leave the other sliced. Roughly chop the almond. Set aside.

Transfer the cooked quinoa to a bowl. Stir in the mashed banana, blueberries, honey, and chia seeds.

Top with sliced banana and chopped almonds.

Nutrition information per serving: Kcal: 306 Protein: 17g, Carbs: 33, Fats: 14g

2.   Flaxseed pancakes with Blueberries and Greek Yogurt

Ingredients:

- 4 eggs, Omega-3 enriched
- 4 tbsp buckwheat flour
- 4 tbsp flax seeds, minced
- 1 cup of almond milk
- ¼ tsp of salt
- 1 cup of Greek yogurt
- 1 cup of fresh blueberries
- Flaxseed oil

Preparation:

Combine the ingredients in a bowl. Beat well with an electric mixer, on high.

Heat up the oil in a medium-sized skillet, over a high temperature. Pour some of the mixture in the skillet and fry the pancakes for about 2-3 minutes, on each side.

This mixture should give you about 8 pancakes. Top each pancake with Greek yogurt and fresh blueberries. Serve.

Nutrition information per serving: Kcal: 161 Protein: 16.5g, Carbs: 10, Fats: 5g

3.   Eggs Stuffed with Shrimps, Avocado and Cress

Ingredients:

- 2 eggs

- 4 small shrimps

- 1 tbsp of Dijon mustard

- ¼ tsp of freshly ground black pepper

- 1 medium-sized avocado, halved

- A handful of finely chopped cress

- Extra virgin olive oil

- ¼ cup of fresh lemon juice

- Fresh lettuce

Preparation:

Heat up two tablespoons of oil over a medium heat. Add shrimps and stir-fry for about five minutes. Remove from the heat and set aside.

Meanwhile, boil the eggs. Gently place two eggs in a pot of boiling water. Cook for 10 minutes. Rinse and drain. Cool for a while and peel. You can add one teaspoon of baking soda in a boiling water. This will make the peeling process much easier.

Cut the eggs in half and remove the yolks.

In a medium-sized bowl, combine the egg yolks with ½ avocado, mustard, black pepper, and lemon juice. Transfer to a blender and pulse to combine. Use this mixture to stuff each egg half.

Top each egg with finely chopped cress and one shrimp. You can add some salt to taste.

Serve with fresh lettuce and chopped avocado.

Nutrition information per serving: Kcal: 170 Protein: 29g, Carbs: 8, Fats: 11g

4.   Greek Yogurt with Muesli, Honey and Kiwi

Ingredients:

- 3.5oz Greek yogurt

- 1 tbsp of honey

- ¼ cup of muesli (I use rolled oats with dried fruits, but any other combination you have on hand will work)

- ½ large banana or 1 small banana, peeled and sliced

- 2 tbsp of raisins

- 2 tbsp of walnuts, finely chopped

Preparation:

Combine the Greek yogurt with honey and mix well with a spoon. Add muesli, sliced banana and top with raisins and finely chopped walnuts.

Serve immediately.

Nutrition information per serving: Kcal: 121 Protein: 19g, Carbs: 16.7g, Fats: 4.5g

5. Spinach Omelet

Ingredients:

- 3 eggs, whole and beaten, Omega-3 enriched
- ½ cup fresh goat's cheese
- ½ cup of onion, peeled and chopped
- 1 cup of fresh spinach, finely chopped
- 2 tbsp of extra virgin olive oil
- salt and pepper, to taste

Preparation:

Heat up the olive oil over a medium temperature. Stir-fry the onions until translucent.

Crack the eggs and mix well with a fork. Add some salt and pepper. Whisk in 1 cup of fresh spinach and ½ cup of cottage cheese. Pour the eggs evenly in a pan and reduce the heat. Cook for about 2 minutes, stirring constantly.

Nutrition information per serving: Kcal: 470, Protein: 32g, Carbs: 9.5g, Fats: 21g

6.   Rolled Oats with Chia Seeds and Flax Seed

Ingredients:

- 5 tbsp of rolled oats

- 1 cup of skim milk

- 1 tbsp of chia seeds

- 1 tbsp of flax seed, minced

- 2 tablespoons of honey

- ½ tsp of raw cocoa

- ¼ tsp of cinnamon, ground

Preparation:

Combine the ingredients (except honey) in a bowl. Add one cup of milk and bring it to a boiling point. Stir well and remove from the heat. Cool for a while and add honey. Let it stand in the refrigerator for about an hour, or even overnight.

Top with fresh fruits and seeds of your choice. Serve cold.

Nutrition information per serving: Kcal: 250 Protein: 15g, Carbs: 35, Fats: 9g

7.   Blueberry Oatmeal with Flaxseed and Almonds

Ingredients:

- 1 cup of rolled oats

- 1 cup of almond milk

- 1/3 cup of blueberries

- ½ tbsp of honey

- ½ tsp powdered vanilla extract

- ¼ tsp of salt

- ¼ tsp of cinnamon

- 2 tbsp of ground flaxseed

- 5-6 almonds, chopped

Preparation:

Combine the oats with almond milk, blueberries, vanilla extract, salt, and cinnamon in a pot. Add about ½ cup of water and bring it to a boil. Reduce the heat and simmer for 5-10 minutes. Remove from the heat and cool for a while. Stir in honey and ground flaxseed. Top with almonds and serve.

Nutrition information per serving: Kcal: 370 Protein: 22g, Carbs: 41, Fats: 17g

8.   Roasted Avocado

Ingredients:

- 3 medium ripe avocados, cut in half

- 6 eggs, Omega-3 enriched

- 1 medium tomato, finely chopped

- 5 tbsp of olive oil

- 2 tsp of dried rosemary

- salt and pepper to taste

Preparation:

Preheat oven to 350 degrees. Cut avocado in half and remove the flesh from the center.

Place one egg and chopped tomato in each avocado half and sprinkle with rosemary, salt and pepper.

Grease the baking pan with olive oil and place the avocados. You want to use a small baking pan so your avocados can fit tightly.

Place in the oven for about 15-20 minutes.

Serve with buckwheat pita bread.

Nutrition information per serving: Kcal: 280, Protein: 28g, Carbs: 41g, Fats: 20g

9.   Vegetarian Lentils

Ingredients:

- 10oz lentils

- 1.5 tbsp of olive oil

- 1 medium-sized carrot, peeled and sliced

- 1 small potato, peeled and chopped

- 1 bay leaf

- ¼ cup of parsley, finely chopped

- ½ tbsp of chili powder

- Salt to taste

Preparation:

Heat up the olive oil in a deep pot. Add sliced carrot, chopped potato and parsley. Mix well and stir-fry for about five minutes on high heat.

Now add the lentils, 1 bay leaf, some salt and chili powder. Add about 4 cups of water and reduce the heat. Cook until lentils soften, for about an hour. Sprinkle with some parsley before serving.

Nutrition information per serving: Kcal: 180, Protein: 10g, Carbs: 25g, Fats: 9g

10. Spiced Pilaf with Saffron

Ingredients:

- Large pinch of good-quality saffron threads
- 16 fl oz boiling water
- 1 tsp salt
- 2 tbsp flaxseed oil
- 2 tbsp olive oil
- 1 large onion, very finely chopped
- 3 tbsp pine kernels
- 12 oz long grain rice
- 2oz sultanas
- 6 green cardamom pods, shells lightly cracked
- 6 cloves
- ¼ tsp of pepper
- Finely chopped fresh coriander or flat-leaved parsley, to garnish

Preparation:

Toast the saffron threads in a dry frying pan over a medium heat, stirring, for 2 minutes, until they give off an aroma.

Immediately tip out onto a plate.

Pour the boiling water into a measuring jug, stir in the saffron and salt and leave to infuse for 30 minutes.

Het up the flaxseed oil and olive oil in a pressure cooker over medium-high heat. Add the onion. With the cooker's lid off, cook for about 5 minutes, stirring constantly.

Lower the heat, stir the pine kernels into the onions and continue cooking for 2 minutes, stirring, until the nuts just begin to turn a golden color.

Stir in the rice, coating all the grains with oil. Stir for 1 minute, then add the sultanas, cardamom pods and cloves. Pour in the saffron-flavored water and bring to a boil. Securely lock the lid and set for 10 minutes on high.

Fluff up the rice and adjust the seasoning. Stir in the herbs and serve.

Nutrition information per serving: Kcal: 361, Protein: 14g, Carbs: 46g, Fats: 10g

11. Lean Brussel Sprouts

Ingredients:

- 1 pound of Brussel sprouts, chopped
- 5 medium sweet potatoes, finely chopped
- 2 red onions, peeled and sliced
- ¼ cup of lime juice
- 1 tbsp of fresh parsley
- 3 tbsp of olive oil

Preparation:

Add 3 tbsp of olive oil in a deep pot. Heat up over a medium-high heat and add onion slices. Cook until translucent, 2-3 minutes.

Add potatoes and Brussel sprouts and reduce the heat. Continue to cook until potatoes soften.

Sprinkle with lemon juice and fresh parsley before serving.

Nutrition information per serving: Kcal: 51, Protein: 7g, Carbs: 22g, Fats: 7g

12.   Beef Stew

Ingredients:

- 2 pounds grass-fed stew beef, boneless
- 1 tbsp extra virgin olive oil
- 6 oz fresh tomato paste
- 2 handfuls baby carrots
- 2 quartered sweet potatoes
- 1 large onion, finely chopped
- 1 handful fresh button mushrooms
- ½ tablespoon salt
- 1 bay leaf
- 2 ½ cups beef broth
- ½ cup fresh green peas
- 1 tsp of dry thyme
- 3 minced garlic cloves

Instructions:

Take a frying pan and set it over high heat. Heat up the olive oil and add beef. Stir-fry the beef on both sides until properly brown. You may have to use more oil depending on how long it takes for meat to brown. Remove from the heat and transfer it to the pressure cooker. In the same pan, fry the onions, turning the heat to medium. Cook the onions for around 5 minutes.

Pour about one cup of water and tomato paste in the frying pan to scoop up any remaining bits of the beef and onions. After this, pour the mixture over the beef in the pressure cooker. Put in all the remaining ingredients and stir properly, especially if the liquid is thick. Toss in the fresh green peas and close the cooker's lid. Set the heat to high and cook for 20 minutes.

13.   Warm Veggies

Ingredients:

- 10oz fresh beans

- 8oz chicken breast, skinless and boneless

- 3 medium-sized tomatoes, finely chopped

- 3 medium-sized onions, peeled and finely chopped

- 2 medium-sized carrots, peeled and sliced

- 2 medium-sized zucchini, peeled and sliced

- 3 tbsp of olive oil

- A handful of finely chopped parsley

- Salt and pepper to taste

Preparation:

Chop the meat into bite-sized pieces. Place in a deep pot. Add the vegetables, olive oil, finely chopped parsley, and some salt and pepper to taste. Pour enough lukewarm water to cover the ingredients. Cover and cook for about an hour over a medium temperature.

SERVING:

Top with some heavy cream, but this is optional.

Nutrition information per serving: Kcal: 165, Protein: 17g, Carbs: 40g, Fats: 9g

14.   Classic Goulash

Ingredients:

- 2 pounds of lean beef, chopped into bite sized pieces
- 3 medium-sized potatoes, peeled and roughly chopped
- 1 small onion, peeled and finely chopped
- 1 large carrot, peeled and sliced
- ½ cabbage head, shredded
- ¼ cup of tomato sauce
- 2 cups of vegetable stock
- ¼ tbsp of chili powder
- Salt and pepper to taste
- Olive oil for frying

Preparation:

Heat up some olive oil in a pressure cooker (about 2-3 tablespoons will be enough). Add the onions and stir fry for several minutes, or until golden brown color.

Now add the tomato paste and stir well again. Cook for several minutes stirring constantly. Then add the meat, chopped potato, sliced carrot and vegetable stock. Bring it to a boil and securely lock the cooker's lid. Set for 45 minutes on high.

Perform a quick release to release the cooker's pressure. Reduce the heat to medium and continue to cook for 15 more minutes.

When the meat has softened, add the cabbage. Season with some salt and pepper to taste and mix well. Cook for about five more minutes and serve!

Nutrition information per serving: Kcal: 271, Protein: 33g, Carbs: 8.5g, Fats: 11.5g

15.   Pumpkin Stew

Ingredients:

- 21oz sweet pumpkin meat, chopped
- 2 medium-sized onions, peeled and finely chopped
- 1 garlic clove
- 1 red pepper, finely chopped
- 1 tbsp of fresh tomato sauce
- ½ tbsp of chili powder
- 2 bay leaves
- 1 cup of water
- 1 tsp of thyme, dry
- Salt and pepper to taste
- Oil for frying

Preparation:

Heat up some oil in a deep pot and add the chopped onions. Stir-fry for two minutes and add finely chopped red pepper, tomato sauce, and chili powder. Continue to fry until the peper has softened. Add the remaining ingredients and cover. Set the heat to minimum and cook for about an hour.

Nutrition information per serving: Kcal: 374, Protein: 27.5g, Carbs: 13.8g, Fats: 23g

16.   Easy White Chili

Ingredients:

- 2 cups of cooked white beans, fresh or canned

- 2 tbsp of all-purpose flour

- 2 tbsp of vegetable ghee

- 1 small onion, chopped

- 1 tbsp of fresh parsley

- 1 tsp of ground chili pepper

- Salt to taste

Preparation:

With the pressure cooker's lid off, melt the vegetable ghee over a high temperature and add onion. Fry for several minutes, or until translucent. Add 2 tbsp of all-purpose flour and stir well for 1 minute.

Now add 2 cups of cooked beans, parsley, chili pepper, and salt. You can use freshly cooked or canned beans. Add some water (enough to cover the beans) and securely lock the cooker's lid. Set for 25 minutes on high.

Nutrition information per serving: Kcal: 287, Protein: 14.6g, Carbs: 30.5g, Fats: 14g

17.   Hot Beans

Ingredients:

- 1 can (14oz) of beans
- 1 can (7oz) sweet corn
- 1 tsp of Tabasco sauce
- 1 tsp of chili powder
- 1 tbsp of chopped parsley
- 3 tbsp of olive oil
- 1 medium-sized onion, peeled and chopped

Preparation:

In a deep pot, heat up the oil over a medium temperature. Stir-fry the onion for a couple of minutes. Add chili pepper and about two tablespoons of water and continue to cook for ten more minutes.

Now add the beans, corn, and about ¼ cup of water. Reduce the heat to medium-low and cover. Cook for about an hour or until beans soften.

Add chopped parsley and Tabasco sauce. This is optional.

COOKING TIP:

You can reduce the cooking time by using pre-cooked beans.

Nutrition information per serving: Kcal: 240, Protein: 17g, Carbs: 34g, Fats: 8g

18.   Warm Beans with Carrots

Ingredients:

- 24oz beans, soaked

- 5 medium-sized carrots

- 2 medium-sized onions, peeled and finely chopped

- 3 garlic cloves, crushed

- 1 small chili pepper, finely chopped

- 1 tbsp of chili powder

- Salt and pepper to taste

- 1 bay leaf

- 3 cups of water

Topping:

- 3 tbsp of all-purpose flour

- 3 tbsp of olive oil

Preparation:

Soak the beans the night before. Rinse well and drain. Set aside.

Heat up one tablespoon of olive oil in a pressure cooker.

Add chopped onions and garlic. Fry for several minutes and add other ingredients. Mix well and securely lock the lid. Set for 20 minutes on high.

Perform a quick release to release the pressure.

Meanwhile, place two tablespoons of olive oil in a frying skillet. Add flour and mix well. Fry for several minutes, or until nice light brown color. Pour the mixture over the beans and serve.

Nutrition information per serving: Kcal: 80, Protein: 9g, Carbs: 10g, Fats: 15g

19.   Grilled Trout with Vegetables

Ingredients:

- 2 pounds of fresh trout
- ½ cup of olive oil
- A handful of fresh parsley
- Several rosemary sprigs
- 1 tbsp of dry mint, ground
- 3 garlic cloves, crushed
- ¼ tsp of red pepper
- Salt to taste

Preparation:

Wash and clean the fish. Cut lengthwise and remove entrails. Combine the olive oil with dry mint, crushed garlic cloves, and red pepper. Brush the fish with this mixture and stuff with fresh parsley and rosemary sprigs.

Preheat the electric grill and fry for about 5-7 minutes on each side.

Nutrition information per serving: Kcal: 123, Protein: 26g, Carbs: 0g, Fats: 1g

20. Chicken Pita with Fresh Vegetables

Ingredients:

- 2 pounds of whole-purpose flour

- 2 tbsp of dry yeast

- 1 tbsp of sugar

- 1 tsp of salt

- 3.5 cups of water

- 1 tbsp of black cumin

Preparation:

Whisk together dry yeast, sugar, salt, and about ¼ cup of warm water. Allow it to stand for about 20 minutes.

Combine the all-purpose flour with the yeast mixture and some water (enough to create a smooth dough). Cover with a cotton cloth and keep it in a warm place for about 40 minutes.

Shape 8 equal bowl and gently press with your hands. Sprinkle with black cumin and bake for 10 minutes at 400 degrees.

For the chicken filling:

8oz chicken breast, boneless and skinless

- 1 medium-sized onion, peeled and finely chopped

- 5 tbsp of olive oil

- 1 tbsp of homemade tomato paste (see the recipe)

- 1 tsp of fresh thyme, finely chopped

- 1 tsp of black cumin

- Salt and pepper to taste

Preparation:

Wash and cut the meat into long, thin strips. Combine the other ingredients in a bowl. Place the meat in it and cover with foil. Allow it to stand for about an hour.

Preheat a non-stick, grill pan over a medium-high temperature. Fry the chicken (with the marinade) for about 10-15 minutes. Stir constantly.

Use this mixture to fill each pita.

Yogurt topping:

Ingredients:

- 1 cup of Greek yogurt

- 1 garlic clove

- 1 tbsp of olive oil

- Salt to taste

Preparation:

Combine the ingredients in a bowl. Keep in the refrigerator and top each pita with this mixture.

Nutrition information per serving: Kcal: 527, Protein: 27.14g, Carbs: 58.69g, Fats: 19.64g

21.   Grilled Platter

Ingredients:

2 pounds of mixed fresh vegetables (tomatoes, red peppers, yellow peppers, onions, eggplant)

For the marinade:

- 2 cups of olive oil
- 5 garlic cloves
- 1 cup of finely chopped parsley
- ¼ cup of fresh thyme
- Salt and pepper to taste

Preparation:

Combine the marinade ingredients in a large bowl. Wash and cut the vegetables and place in the marinade. Let it stand for 20 minutes.

Preheat an electric grill over a medium-high temperature. Grill for several minutes.

Nutrition information per serving: Kcal: 162, Protein: 3g, Carbs: 12g, Fats: 10g

22.   Kefir Meatballs

Ingredients:

- 1 pound of minced meat (70% beef brisket and 30% lamb shoulder)
- 1 large onion, peeled and finely chopped
- 1 tbsp of finely chopped, fresh rosemary
- 1 whole egg
- ¼ cup of kefir cream
- Salt and pepper to taste
- About 2 tbsp of whole-purpose flour
- Oil

For the topping:

- 2 cups of kefir
- 3 garlic cloves, crushed
- 1 tbsp of fresh rosemary, finely chopped
- Salt to taste

Preparation:

Combine the ingredients in a large bowl. Add about two tablespoons of oil in the mixture and shape the meatballs using your hands.

Heat up some oil in a large skillet, over a medium-high temperature. Fry the meatballs for about 10 minutes, or until lightly charred. Remove from the heat and allow it to cool.

Combine two cups of kefir with crushed garlic and fresh rosemary. Top the meatballs with it.

These meatballs are best cold. I suggest you keep them in the refrigerator overnight.

Nutrition information per serving: Kcal: 60, Protein: 11.5g, Carbs: 10g, Fats: 7g

23.   Grilled Sea Bream

Ingredients:

- 1 medium-sized sea bream
- 1 cup of olive oil
- ½ lemon, sliced
- ¼ cup of lemon juice
- 1 tsp of dry rosemary, ground
- 1 tbsp of fresh parsley, finely chopped
- 3 garlic cloves, crushed
- ¼ tsp of sea salt

Preparation:

Wash and pat dry the fish using a kitchen paper.

Combine the olive oil, lemon juice, dry rosemary, fresh parsley, crushed garlic cloves, and sea salt in a large bowl. Soak the fish in this marinate and leave in the refrigerator for at least 30 minutes (it can stand in the refrigerator up to 2 hours).

Meanwhile, preheat a grill pan over a medium-high temperature.

Remove the fish from the refrigerator and grill for about 10 minutes. Add some of the marinade while grilling (one or two tablespoons at a time).

Nutrition information per serving: Kcal: 103, Protein: 16.7g, Carbs: 0g, Fats: 4g

24. Fresh Lentil Soup

Ingredients:

- 2 spring onions, finely chopped

- 2 carrots, sliced

- 6oz lentils, soaked

- ½ tsp salt

- ¼ tsp pepper

- 3 tbsp sour cream

- Vegetable oil

Preparation:

Soak the lentils for about one hour before cooking.

Heat up the olive oil over a medium temperature in a deep pot. Add spring onions and stir-fry for 2 minutes. Now add sliced carrots. Season with salt and pepper and continue to cook for 3-4 minutes, stirring constantly.

Add lentils, pour 4 cups of water and reduce the heat. Cook for about 20 minutes or until lentils soften. Top with sour cream before serving.

Nutrition information per serving: Kcal: 186, Protein: 10.5g, Carbs: 26.5g, Fats: 4.5g

25.   Carrot Soup

Ingredients:

- 5 large carrots, sliced

- 1 cup of vegetable broth

- 2 cups of water

- ¼ tsp of sea salt

- 1 tsp of dry rosemary

Preparation:

Combine the ingredients in a deep pot. Set the heat to medium-high and bring it to a boil. Reduce the heat to low and continue to cook for 12 minutes. Serve.

Nutrition information per serving: Kcal: 95, Protein: 6g, Carbs: 14.5g, Fats: 2g

26.   Autumn Soup

Ingredients:

- 3 medium-sized sweet potatoes, sliced
- 1 tsp of sea salt
- ¼ tsp of vanilla extract
- 2 fennel bulbs, sliced
- 15 ounces pureed pumpkin
- 1 large onion, sliced
- 1 tbsp of coconut oil
- 5 cups of water

Preparation:

Melt the coconut oil in a deep pot. Turn the heat to high and add onion and fennel bulbs. Cook for 3-5 minutes. Add other ingredients and reduce the heat. Cover and continue to cook for 10-15 minutes. Transfer the soup to a food processor and mix well for 20 seconds.

SERVING:

Top with 1 tablespoon of sour cream before serving.

Nutrition information per serving: Kcal: 129, Protein: 5g, Carbs: 22g, Fats: 3g

27.   Pumpkin Leek Soup

Ingredients:

- 2 leeks, washed and trimmed
- 2 pounds pumpkin, chopped and peeled
- ¼ tsp black pepper, ground
- 1 tsp sea salt
- 1 teaspoon ginger, grated
- 1 garlic clove, crushed
- 3 cups chicken broth
- 2 tablespoons olive oil
- 1 teaspoon cumin
- 1 teaspoon ginger powder

Preparation:

Heat the olive oil in a deep pot. Add chopped leeks, garlic, and enough water to cover. Cook until leeks soften.

Pour ginger powder and cumin over the leeks to season them. Fry for one more minute.

Add other ingredients and mix well. Reduce the heat and cook for 12 minutes.

Nutrition information per serving: Kcal: 167, Protein: 9g, Carbs: 32g, Fats: 3g

28.   Simple Bean Soup

Ingredients:

- 1 cup of fresh beans, pre-cooked

- 3 cups of water

- ¼ tsp of sea salt

- 1 tsp of dry mint

Preparation:

Combine the ingredients in a blender and pulse for 30 seconds. Transfer to a deep pot and add two cups of water. Bring it to a boil and reduce the heat. Cook for 5-7 minutes.

Nutrition information per serving: Kcal: 137, Protein: 6.5g, Carbs: 19g, Fats: 4g

29. Avocado and Mint Soup

Ingredients:

- 3 tbsp extra virgin olive oil

- 6 spring onions, sliced

- 1 garlic clove, crushed

- 4 tbsp plain flour

- 3 cups of vegetable stock

- 2 ripe avocados

- 2-3 tsp lemon juice

- Pinch of grated lemon zest

- 5 floz milk

- 5 floz single cream

- 1-1½ tbsp chopped fresh mint

- Salt and pepper

- Sprigs of fresh mint, for garnish

Preparation:

Heat up the olive oil in a deep pot. Add sliced onions and garlic. Stir-fry for about 3 minutes, or until translucent.

Now add flour and cook for about one more minute.

Slowly add the stock and bring it to a boil. Reduce the heat to miminum and continue to cook.

Meanwhile, prepare the avocados – peel and remove the core. Chop into bite-sized pieces. Transfer to a pot. Cover and simmer for ten more minutes.

Remove the pot from the heat and cool for a while. Transfer to a food processor and blend until smooth.

Stir in some milk, cream, lemon zest, lemon juice, and mint.

Serve.

Nutrition information per serving: Kcal: 109, Protein: 2g, Carbs: 7.5g, Fats: 8g

30.   Avocado and Vegetable Soup

Ingredients:

- 1 large, ripe avocado
- 2 tbsp lemon juice
- 1 tbsp vegetable oil
- 4½ oz canned sweetcorn, drained
- 2 tomatoes, skinned and deseeded
- 1 garlic clove, crushed
- 1 leek, chopped
- 1 red chilli, chopped
- 14 floz vegetable stock
- 5 floz milk
- Shredded leek, to garnish

Preparation:

Peel the avocado and mash the flesh with a fork, stir in the lemon juice and reserve until required.

Heat the oil in a large saucepan. Add the sweetcorn, tomatoes, garlic, lee and chilli and saute over a low heat for 2-3 minutes or until softened.

Put half of the vegetable mixture in a food processor and blender, add the mashed avocado and process until smooth. Transfer the contents to a clean saucepan.

Add the vegetable stock, milk and reserved vegetables and cook over a low heat for 3-4 minutes until hot. Transfer to warmed individual serving bowls, garnish with shredded leek and serve immediately.

Tip:

If serving chilled, transfer from the food processor to a bowl, and stir in the vegetable stock, milk and reserved vegetables. Cover and refrigerate for at least 4 hours.

Nutrition information per serving: Kcal: 167 Protein: 4g, Carbs: 8g, Fats: 13g

31.   Curried Parsnip Soup

Ingredients:

- 2 tbsp vegetable oil

- 1 red onion, chopped

- 3 parsnips, chopped

- 2 garlic cloves, crushed

- 2 tspgaram masala

- ½ tsp chili powder

- 1 tbsp plain flour

- 5 floz vegetable stock

- Grated rind and juice of 1 lemon

- Salt and pepper

- Strips of lemon rind, to garnish

Preparation:

Heat the oil in a large saucepan. Add the onion, parsnips and garlic and saute, stirring frequently, for 5-7 minutes until the vegetables have softened but not changed color.

Add the garam masala and chili powder and cook, stirring constantly, for 30 seconds. Sprinkle in the flour, mix well and cook, stirring constantly, for another 30 seconds.

Stir in the stock, lemon rind and lemon juice and bring to a boil. Lower the heat and simmer for 20 minutes.

Remove some of the vegetable pieces with a slotted spoon and reserve until required. Process the remaining soup and vegetables in a food processor or blender for about 1 minute to a smooth puree.   Alternatively, put the vegetables in a sieve and press through with the back of a wooden spoon.

Return the soup to a clean saucepan and stir in the reserved vegetables. Heat the soup through for 2 minutes until piping hot.

Season to taste with salt and pepper then transfer to soup bowls. Garnish with strips of lemon and serve.

Nutrition information per serving: Kcal: 152 Protein: 3g, Carbs: 10g, Fats: 8g

32.   Vichyssoise

Ingredients:

- 3 large leeks

- 3 tbsp olive oil

- 1 onion, thinly sliced

- 1 lb 2oz potatoes, chopped

- 1½ pints vegetable stock

- 2 tsp lemon juice

- Pinch of ground nutmeg

- ¼ tsp ground coriander

- 1 bay leaf

- 1 egg yolk

- 5 floz single cream

- Salt and white pepper

- Freshly snipped chives, to garnish

Preparation:

First you will have to prepare the leeks. Trim the ends and finely chop.

Heat um the olive oil in a medium-sized skillet and add

leeks. Add the onion and stir-fry for a couple of minutes, or until translucent.

Now add chopped potatoes, stock, lemon juice, coriander, nutmeg, lemon juice, and bay leaf. Season with some salt and pepper and bring it to a boil. Reduce the heat to miminum and simmer for 25-30 minutes.

Remove from the heat and cool for a while. Transfer to a food processor and blend until smooth.

Now gently whisk in the egg and cream. Mix well and gently reheat.

Sprinlke with chives and serve.

Nutrition information per serving: Kcal: 208 Protein: 5g, Carbs: 20g, Fats: 12g

33.   Tomato and Red Pepper Soup

Ingredients:

- 2 large red peppers

- 1 large onion, chopped

- 2 celery sticks, trimmed and chopped

- 1 garlic clove, crushed

- 1 pint fresh vegetable stock

- 2 bay leaves

- 1 lb 12 oz canned plum tomatoes

- Salt and pepper

- 2 spring onions, finely shredded, to garnish

- Fresh crusty bread, to serve

Preparation:

Preheat the grill to hot. Halve and deseed the red peppers, arrange them on the grill rack and cook, turning occasionally, for 8-10 minutes until softened and charred.

Let the red peppers cool slightly, then carefully peel off the charred skins. Reserve a small piece of red pepper flesh for garnish, chop the rest and place in a large saucepan.

Mix in the onion, celery and garlic. Add the stock and bay leaves. Bring to a boil, cover and simmer for about 15 minutes. Remove from heat.

Lift out the bay leaves from the pan and discard them. Stir in the tomatoes and then transfer to a blender. Process for a few seconds until smooth. Return to the pan.

Season to taste and heat for about 3-4 minutes until piping hot. Ladle into warm bowls and garnish with the reserved red pepper cut into strips and the spring onions. Serve with fresh crusty bread.

Tip:

If you prefer a coarser, more robust soup, lightly mash the tomatoes with a wooden spoon and omit the blending process.

Nutrition information per serving: Kcal: 52 Protein: 3g, Carbs: 10g, Fats: 0.4g

34.   Grilled Squid with Swiss Chard

Ingredients:

- 1 pound of fresh squid

- Olive oil

- Salt to taste

- 1 tsp of dry rosemary

Preparation:

Wash and pat dry the squids. Remove the heads and clean each squid.

In a small bowl, combine the olive oil with dry rosemary, and salt. Mix well to combine. Use a kitchen brush to spread this mixture over the squids. Allow it to stand for about 15 minutes.

Preheat the grill pan over medium-high temperature. Fry the squids for several minutes on each side. Serve immediately!

Swiss chard

Ingredients:

- 1 pound of Swiss chard

- 1 medium-sized potato

- ½ cup of olive oil

- Salt to taste

- Water

Preparation:

Rinse the Swiss chard and transfer to a deep pot. Add enough water to cover and briefly boil (for about five minutes). Remove from the heat and drain. Set aside.

Peel and chop the potato in small cubes. Pour the olive oil in a deep, large pot, and add about 1 cup of water. Place the potato in it and cook until soft. This should take about 15 minutes. Now add the Swiss chard, mix well and cook for 10 more minutes. Serve.

Nutrition information per serving: Kcal: 105, Protein: 12.9g, Carbs: 11.8g, Fats: 1.1g

35.   Braised Leeks with Beef

Ingredients:

- 6 large leeks
- 1 pound of lean beef meat
- 1 bay leaf
- 1 carrot, sliced
- Large handful of chopped celery
- 1 small onion, peeled and sliced
- ¼ tsp of pepper
- Pinch of salt
- 3 tbsp of extra virgin olive oil
- 2 tbsp of vegetable oil
- ¼ cup of white wine
- ½ tsp of dry rosemary

Preparation:

Grease the bottom of your pressure cooker with 2 tablespoons of vegetable oil. Season the meat with some salt and pepper. Place in your cooking pot. Add sliced onion, carrot, celery, and 1 bay leaf. Pour enough water to cover and seal the lid. Bring the cooker up to full pressure and reduce to minimum. Cook for 45 minutes. Remove from the heat and set aside.

Trim the leeks and remove the first two layers. Chop into bite-sized pieces. Heat up the olive oil over medium-high temperature and stir-fry the leeks for several minutes.

Remove the meat from the cooking pot. Chop into smaller pieces and add to the frying skillet. Add ¼ cup of white wine, dry rosemary, and some salt to taste. Cook for another 10-12 minutes.

Nutrition information per serving: Kcal: 420, Protein: 19g, Carbs: 25g, Fats: 27g

You can use the beef stock to prepare a soup. Pour into a deep cooking pot and bring it to a boil. Add a handful of soup noodles, one tablespoon of chopped parsley and cook for about 3-4 minutes. Serve warm.

Nutrition information per serving: Kcal: 79, Protein: 6g, Carbs: 10g, Fats: 2g

36.   Grilled Turkey with Boiled Potatos and Olive Oil

Ingredients:

- 0.5oz turkey breast, boneless and skinless

- 1 cup of olive oil

- 4 cloves of garlic

- 2 tbsp apple vinegar

- 5 tbsp fresh parsley, finely chopped

- 1 tsp oregano, dry

- ½ tsp salt

Preparation:

Wash and pat dry the meat. Set aside.

Combine all the other ingredients in a large bowl. Place the meat in it and marinate for about an hour.

Preheat the grill pan and grill the meat for about 10 minutes on each side. You can add some marinade while frying (1 tbsp will be enough).

You can serve it with boiled potato and broccoli. Peel the potato and slice into thin slices. Transfer to a deep pot and add enough water to cover. Cook until each slice softens.

Remove from the heat and drain. Allow it to cool for a while.

Meanwhile, repeat the process with broccoli. They take about 10 minutes to soften. Combine the potato with broccoli, season with some salt and olive oil.

This recipe is almost impossible without garlic. 1 crushed garlic clove will be enough. Combine it with olive oil, add 1 tbsp of finely chopped parsley and pour over vegetables.

Nutrition information per serving: Kcal: 153, Protein:34g, Carbs: 0g, Fats: 0.8g

37.　White Buzzara Mussels

Ingredients:

- 2 pounds of fresh mussels
- 3 cloves of garlic, crushed
- 2oz breadcrumbs
- ½ cup of white wine
- ½ cup of olive oil
- Handful of finely chopped parsley
- ½ lemon

Preparation:

Wash and rinse each mussel.

Preheat the olive oil over medium-high temperature, in a large and deep pot. Add crushed garlic and stir-fry for about a minute.

Transfer the mussels in a cooking pot, add wine, finely chopped parsley, breadcrumbs, and cover. Cook for about 15 minutes, or until mussels open.

Nutrition information per serving: Kcal: 101, Protein: 19.4, Carbs: 1.3g, Fats: 1.5g

38.   Buckwheat Pasta with Homemade Tomato Sauce

Ingredients:

- 1 pack of buckwheat pasta

- 3 large ripe tomatoes

- 1 tbsp of olive oil

- 2 garlic cloves, crushed

- ½ tsp of dry oregano

- ¼ tsp of salt

- 1 tsp of sugar

Preparation:

Use the package instructions to prepare pasta. Rinse well and drain. Set aside.

Peel and roughly chop the tomatoes. Make sure you keep all the liquid.

Heat up the olive oil over a medium temperature. Add the garlic and stir-fry for several minutes. Now add tomatoes, oregano, salt, sugar, and oregano. Reduce the heat to low and cook until the tomatoes have softened. Add ¼ cup of water and cook for 10 more minutes stirring constantly. Turn off the heat, add pasta and cover. Let it stand for 10 minutes before serving.

Serve it with grated smoked cheese, grated Parmesan, crushed garlic, finely chopped parsley, or whatever you like.

Nutrition information per serving: Kcal: 293, Protein: 9.87g, Carbs: 53.62g, Fats: 3.99g

39.   Seafood Risotto

Ingredients:

- 1 cup of brown rice
- 8oz fres seafood mix
- ½ cup of peas, cooked
- 1 small tomato
- ½ bell pepper, finely chopped
- 1 tbsp of ground turmeric
- Salt to taste

Preparation:

Briefly boil the seafood mix, for about 3-4 minutes. Drain and set aside.

Add one cup of rice and 3 cups of water in a deep pot. Bring it to a boil and cook for about 10 minutes, or until half of the water has evaporated.

Meanwhile, peel and finely chop the tomato and bell pepper. Mix with peas in a bowl and season with salt.

Combine this mixture with rice, add seafood mix, one tablespoon of ground turmeric and cook until all the water has evaporated. You can serve with some grated Parmesan cheese.

Nutrition information per serving: Kcal: 379, Protein:22.85, Carbs: 40.03g, Fats: 13.06g

40.   Salmon Cannelloni

Ingredients:

- 1 pack of cannelloni (8.8oz)

- 3 tbsp extra virgin olive oil

- 3oz all-purpose flour

- 2pts milk

- 8.8oz ricotta cheese

- 3oz grated Parmesan cheese

- 5oz smoked salmon, thinly sliced

- Seasoning to taste

Preparation:

Bring the olive oil, flour and milk slowly to a boil, whisking constantly until thickened. Put half of the sauce into a bowl and mix with ricotta, parmesan, salmon, and seasoning to taste. Use to fill the cannelloni and arrange in a baking dish. Cover with remaining white sauce and place in the oven for 40 minutes, or until golden brown.

Nutrition information per serving: Kcal: 351, Protein:24, Carbs: 42g, Fats: 17g

41.   Cabbage Rolls with Turkey and Rice

Ingredients:

- 1 pound of fresh cabbage leaves
- 1 medium turkey fillet, boneless and skinless
- ½ cup of rice, cooked
- 1 medium tomato
- 1 tbsp of fresh parsley, chopped
- ¼ tsp of sea salt
- ¼ tsp of black pepper, ground
- 5 tbsp of olive oil

Preparation:

Wash and pat dry the meat. Using a sharp knife, cut the meat into small pieces. If this sounds like too much work, you can simply use minced turkey fillets.

Wash, peel and finely chop the tomato. Place it in a large bowl. Combine with the meat, rice, parsley, salt and pepper. Add about two tablespoons of olive oil to this mixture. Place about two tablespoons of this mixture in the center of each cabbage leaf. Roll up nicely tuck in the ends.

Now add the remaining oil in a deep pot. Carefully place

the rolls in a pot and add about 1 cup of water. Cover and cook over a minimum temperature for about an hour.

Nutrition information per serving: Kcal: 117, Protein:8.81g, Carbs: 8.97g, Fats: 5.31g

42.   Fish Stew with Homemade Polenta

Ingredients:

- 1 cup of diced fire roasted tomatoes
- 2 pound of mixed fish (mackerel, whiting fish, salmon)
- 1 tbsp of dried basil
- 6 cups of fish stock
- Salt and pepper to taste
- 6 tbsp of homemade tomato paste
- 6 chopped celery stalks
- 3 chopped carrots
- ½ cup of olive oil
- 1 finely chopped onion
- 6 garlic cloves, crushed
- ½ cup of button mushrooms

Preparation:

Heat up the olive oil in a frying pan, over a medium temperature. Add chopped celery, onions, and carrots. Stir well and fry for about 10 minutes. Remove from the heat and transfer to a deep pot. Add the remaining ingredients and cook for about 15 minutes, over a medium temperature.

Homemade polenta

Ingredients:

- 17oz corn flour

- 5 cups of water

- 5 tbsp of olive oil

- A pinch of salt

Preparation:

Bring five cups of water to a boiling point. Add salt, olive oil, and reduce the heat to medium. Slowly whisk in the corn flour. Cook until the mixture thickens, stirring often. Remove from the heat and serve.

Nutrition information per serving: Kcal: 128, Protein: 1.7g, Carbs: 15.3g, Fats: 6.9g

43.   Boiled Potatoes with Olive Oil

Ingredients:

- 2 medium-sized potatoes, boiled

- 5 spring onions, finely chopped

- 1 small red onion, peeled and sliced

- Olive oil to taste

- Salt to taste

- Pepper to taste

Preparation:

First you will have to boil the potatoes. Peel and thoroughly rinse the potatoes. Slice and transfer to a deep pot. Add just enough water to cover. Bring it to a boil and cook for about 15 minutes, or until the potatoes have softened. Remove from the heat and drain. Allow it to cool for a while.

Meanwhile, prepare the onions. Trim the roots away and strip off any extra outer leaves. Finely chop and combine with potatoes.

Peel and slice the onion. Add to the salad mixture. Season with olive oil, salt and pepper to taste. You can add a few drops of fresh lemon juice, but this is optional.

Serve cold.

Nutrition information per serving: Kcal: 357, Protein: 7g, Carbs: 28g, Fats: 20g

44.   Greek Octopus

Ingredients:

- 1 pound of fresh octopus

- 1 small onion, finely chopped

- Few ripe cherry tomatoes

- Few black and green olives

- 1 tbsp of capers

- ¼ cup of olive oil

- 1 tbsp of finely chopped parsley

- Salt to taste

Preparation:

Place the octopus in a pressure cooker. Add 2 cups of water and seal the lid. Cook for about 40-45 minutes. Remove from the heat and allow it to cool for a while. Slice the octopus into bite-sized pieces and set aside.

Preheat two tablespoons of olive oil in a large skillet. Add the onions and stir-fry for five minutes. Now add parsley and octopus. Mix well and fry for about five more minutes. Remove from the heat and transfer to a bowl. Add halved cherry tomatoes, olives, capers, and season with the remaining olive oil and salt.

Keep it in the refrigerator for at least an hour before serving.

You can serve this salad with some boiled potatoes, Swiss chard, or leeks.

Nutrition information per serving: Kcal: 188, Protein: 20.7g, Carbs: 5.6g, Fats: 8.9g

45. Seafood Pasta

Ingredients:

- 1 pack of buckwheat pasta
- 1 pound of fresh seafood mix
- 4 tbsp of olive oil
- 2 garlic cloves, crushed
- 1 small onion, peeled and finely chopped
- ½ tsp of dry oregano
- ¼ tsp of salt

Preparation:

Use the package instructions to prepare pasta. Rinse well and drain. Set aside.

Heat up the olive oil over a medium temperature. Add the onion and garlic and stir-fry for several minutes, or until translucent. Now add seafood mix, oregano, and salt. Reduce the heat to low and cook until the seafood mix have softened. You might want to check the octopus as it takes the most time to soften.

Turn off the heat, add pasta and cover. Let it stand for 10 minutes before serving.

46.   Spring Lentils with Olive Oil

Ingredients:

- 1 cup of cooked lentils

- 2 boiled eggs

- 1 small eggplant

- 1 large red onion

- ½ cup of green onions, chopped

- ¼ cup of low fat cream

- ¼ cup of lemon juice

- 2 tbsp of olive oil

- 1 tbsp of chopped parsley

Preparation:

First you have to cook your lentils. Use 3 cups of water for 1 cup of dry lentils. Cooked lentils will double in size. Keep this in mind when cooking. Bring the water to a boiling point, reduce the heat to medium and cover. Cook for about 15-20 minutes. Remove from the heat and drain.

Peel and wash the eggplant. Cut into thin slices and combine with a low fat cream, lemon juice and olive oil. Use an electric mixer, or a blender to get a smooth mousse.

Allow it to cool in the refrigerator for about 30 minutes. Meanwhile cut the vegetables into thin slices. Mix with lentils and eggplant mousse. Sprinkle with some parsley and serve.

Nutrition information per serving: Kcal: 252, Protein: 34.5g, Carbs: 47g, Fats: 13g

47. Grilled Shrimps with Broccoli

Ingredients:

- 1 pound of frozen shrimps
- ½ pound of fresh broccoli
- Vegetable oil
- Salt to taste

Preparation:

Heat up some olive oil in a deep frying skillet, over a high temperature. Place the shrimps in it and fry for several minutes. You want them to be nice and crispy.

Remove from the heat and use some kitchen paper to soak up the excess oil. Now add the broccoli in the same skillet and fry for about 5 more minutes. Transfer to a plate and sprinkle with some salt. Serve immediately.

Nutrition information per serving: Kcal: 224, Protein: 27.1g, Carbs: 10g, Fats: 5g

48.   Meatballs with Onions and Rosemary

Ingredients:

- 1 pound of minced meat (70% beef brisket and 30% lamb shoulder)
- 1 large onion, peeled and finely chopped .
- 1 tbsp of finely chopped, fresh rosemary
- 1 whole egg
- Salt and pepper to taste
- About 2 tbsp of rice flour
- Oil

Preparation:

Combine the ingredients in a large bowl. Add about two tablespoons of oil in the mixture and shape the meatballs using your hands.

Heat up some oil in a large skillet, over a medium-high temperature. Fry the meatballs for about 10 minutes, or until lightly charred. Remove from the heat and serve.

Nutrition information per serving: Kcal: 57, Protein: 3.47g, Carbs: 2.12, Fats: 3.69g

49.   Lentil Salad

Ingredients:

- 1 cup of cooked lentils
- 1 medium-sized red bell pepper
- ½ cup of sweet corn
- A handful of purple cabbage, shredded
- A handful of lettuce, shredded
- ½ tsp of salt
- ¼ tsp of black pepper, freshly ground
- 2 tbsp of olive oil
- 1 tbsp of sesame seeds

Preparation:

First you have to cook your lentils. Use 3 cups of water for 1 cup of dry lentils. Cooked lentils will double in size. Keep this in mind when cooking. Bring the water to a boiling point, reduce the heat to medium and cover. Cook for about 15-20 minutes. Remove from the heat and drain. Transfer to a bowl.

Now add other ingredients, season with salt, pepper, olive oil, and sprinkle with sesame seeds. Toss well to combine.

Nutrition information per serving: Kcal: 184 Protein: 23g, Carbs: 27g, Fats: 11g

50.   Greek Salad

Ingredients:

- 1 cup of fresh goat's cheese

- 1 whole egg, bolied

- ½ cup of red cabbage, shredded

- Few lettuce leaves

- 1 small tomato, chopped

- 1 small onion, peeled and sliced

- ½ cucumber, peeled and sliced

- ½ red bell pepper, sliced

- Few olives

- 1 small chili pepper

- ¼ cup of olive oil

- 1 tsp of mustard

- 1 tbsp of finely chopped parsley

- 1 garlic clove, crushed

- ¼ tsp of sea salt

- Black pepper to taste

Preparation:

Combine the olive oil with mustard, finely chopped parsley, and one garlic clove. Season with some salt and pepper and mix well.

Place the vegetables on a serving plate. Drizzle with the olive oil dressing and serve immediately.

Nutrition information per serving: Kcal: 299 Protein: 35g, Carbs: 22g, Fats: 26g

51.   Wild Asparagus with Tuna and Garlic

Ingredients:

- 8oz fresh, wild asparagus

- 1 (12oz)tuna steak

- 2 cloves of garlic

- 2 tbsp of vegetable oil, for frying

- ¼ tsp of freshly ground white pepper

- 4 tbsp of extra virgin olive oil

- ¼ tsp of salt

- Black olives for decoration

Preparation:

Heat up two tablespoons of extra virgin olive oil over a medium-high temperature. Season the tuna steak with some salt and white pepper. Cook for five minutes on each side.

Remove from the skillet and cool for a while. Flake the tuna steak into small pieces.

Clean and cut the asparagus into 2 inch long strips. Heat up 2 tbsp of olive oil over a medium-high temperature. Add asparagus and stir-fry for several minutes. Remove from the heat and use some kitchen paper to soak the excess oil. Transfer to a serving platter and top with tuna. Season with some salt and top with black olives.

Nutrition information per serving: Kcal: 160 Protein: 18g, Carbs: 16.5g, Fats: 11g

52.   Crispy Beans with Lime

Ingredients:

- ½ red onion, peeled and sliced

- 2oz of green beans, cooked

- 3 cherry tomatoes, halved

- 3 slices of red bell pepper

For dressing:

- ¼ cup of fresh lime juice

- 3 tbsp of olive oil

- 1 tsp of honey

- ½ small shallot, minced

- 1 garlic clove, crushed

- ¼ tsp of salt

Preparation:

Combine the lime juice with honey. Mix well with a fork. Slowly add the olive oil, whisking constantly. Now add the minced shallot, crushed garlic clove, and salt. Set aside.

Combine the ingredients in a medium-sized bowl. Add the

dressing and toss well to combine. Serve cold.

Nutrition information per serving: Kcal: 141 Protein: 3.5g, Carbs: 21g, Fats: 6.5g

53.   Grilled Chicken Salad

Ingredients:

- 2 pieces of chicken breast, boneless and skinless
- ¼ cup of silken tofu, sliced
- 1 cup of lamb's lettuce
- 1 cup of cherry tomatoes
- ½ cup of button mushrooms, sliced
- 1 small zucchini, chopped
- ¼ tsp of salt
- 1/5 tsp of red pepper, ground
- 2 tbsp of olive oil

Preparation:

Wash and pat dry the meat with some kitchen paper. Cut into bite size pieces. Peel and chop the zucchini.

I like to prepare this salad in a large grill pan. Heat up some olive oil over high temperature and add chopped chicken meat. Stir well and fry for about 5-10 minutes. Now add sliced zuccini and mushrooms. Stir well again and cook for five more minutes. Remove from the heat and allow it to cool for a while.

Meanwhile, cut cherry tomatoes in half and combine with lamb's lettuce and silken tofu. Add chicken mix and season with salt and red pepper.

Nutrition information per serving: Kcal: 233 Protein: 26g, Carbs: 15g, Fats: 11g

54.   Lettuce Salad with Walnuts

Ingredients:

- 2 cups of lettuce, chopped

- 1 large orange

- ¼ cup of walnuts

- ¼ cup of dates, finely chopped

- 1 tbsp of fresh lemon juice

Preparation:

Combine the ingredients in a large bowl and season with lemon juice. Mix well and serve cold.

Nutrition information per serving: Kcal: 148 Protein: 12g, Carbs: 21g, Fats: 8.3g

55.   Wild Salmon Salad with Lettuce and Fresh Lime

Ingredients:

- 10oz wild salmon fillets, boneless

- 1 bay leaf

- 7oz lettuce, torn

- 1 medium-sized cucumber, sliced

- 2 boiled eggs

- ½ cup of fat-free sour cream

- 1 tbsp Dijon mustard

- 1 tbsp extra virgin olive oil

- 2 tbsp fresh lime juice

- ½ tsp of salt

Preparation:

Place the salmon fillets in a pot. Add bay leaf and enough water to cover. Bring it to a boil and reduce the heat. Cook for 10 minutes. Remove from the heat, drain and chop into bite-sized pieces.

Meanwhile, boil the eggs. Gently place two eggs in a pot of boiling water. You can add one teaspoon of baking soda to make the peeling process easier. Cook for 7-10 minutes.

Rinse and cool for a while. Peel the eggs, slice and transfer to a plate. Add sliced cucumber and chopped salmon. Set aside.

In a small bowl, combine sour cream with Dijon, extra virgin olive oil, fresh lime juice, and salt. Drizzle over salad and serve.

Nutrition information per serving: Kcal: 350, Protein: 27.5g, Carbs: 16g, Fats: 19.5g

56.   Chickpea Salad

Ingredients:

- ½ cup of cooked lentils

- ½ cup of cooked chickpeas

- ½ red onion, finely chopped

- 1 cup of lettuce, finely chopped

- 3 tbsp of fresh lemon juice

- 2 tbsp of olive oil

Preparation:

First you will have to cook the lentils. For ½ cup of dry lentils, you will need 1 ½ cup of water, because the lentils will double in size. Bring it to a boil, reduce the heat and cook for about 15-20 minutes, or until the lentils have softened. Remove from the heat and drain. Allow it to cool for a while.

Place all the ingredients in a bowl and mix well. Before serving, add three tablespoons of fresh lemon juice and two tablespoons of olive oil. Toss well to coat.

Nutrition information per serving: Kcal: 249, Protein: 8g, Carbs: 26g, Fats: 14g

57.   Italian Seafood Salad

Ingredients:

- Fresh lettuce leaves, rinsed

- 1 small cucumber sliced

- ½ red bell pepper, sliced

- 1 cup of fresh seafood mix

- 1 onion, peeled and finely chopped

- 3 garlic cloves, crushed

- ¼ cup of fresh orange juice

- 5 tbsp of extra virgin olive oil

- Salt to taste

Preparation:

Heat up 3 tbsp of extra virgin olive oil over medium-high temperature. Add chopped onion and crushed garlic. Stir fry for about 5 minutes. Reduce the heat to minimum and add 1 cup of frozen seafood mix. Cover and cook for about 15 minutes, until soft. Remove from the heat and allow it to cool for a while.

Meanwhile, combine the vegetables in a bowl. Add the remaining 2 tbsp of olive oil, fresh orange juice and little salt. Toss well to combine.

Top with seafood mix and serve immediately.

Nutrition information per serving: Kcal: 170 Protein: 17g, Carbs: 4g, Fats: 11g

58.   Spring Salad

Ingredients:

- ½ cup of lettuce, finely chopped
- ½ cup of sweet corn
- 1 red bell pepper, sliced
- ½ green bell pepper, sliced
- 5 cherry tomatoes, halved
- ½ red onion, peeled and sliced
- 1 tsp of dry rosemary, crushed
- Few drops of fresh lime juice

Preparation:

Wash and cut the bell peppers in half. Remove the seeds and the pulp. Slice into thin slices.

Peel and slice the onion.

Use a big serving platter and arrange the vegetables. You can play with some colors, or even add some ingredients you like. Sprinkle with some rosemary and fresh lime juice. Serve immediately.

Nutrition information per serving: Kcal: 35, Protein: 3g, Carbs: 7g, Fats: 1g

112 Sleep Improving Juice and Meal Recipes

59.   Light Banana Dessert

Ingredients:

- 1 large banana

- 1 tbsp of maple syrup

- 1 tbsp of low fat whipped dessert topping

- 1 tbsp of fat free cocoa dessert topping

Preparation:

Peel and cut the banana into bite size pieces. Trasfer to a serving bowl. Gently whisk together maple syrup and dessert topping and pour over banana. Sprinke some cocoa on top. Serve cold.

Nutrition information per serving: Kcal: 287, Protein: 13g, Carbs: 51g, Fats: 4g

60. Blueberry Muffins

Ingredients:

- 2 cups of all purpose flour
- 1 tbsp of baking powder
- ½ tsp of salt
- ½ cup of sugar
- 1 cup of milk
- ½ cup of water
- 2 eggs
- ¼ cup of canola oil
- ½ cup of fresh blueberries
- muffin molds

Preparation:

Preheat oven to 350 degrees.

Mix all dry ingredients in a large bowl. Whisk in eggs, canola oil, sugar, milk and water. Mix well with an electric mixer. Now add blueberries and mix again. Shape muffins with this mixture using muffin molds. Transfer to a baking sheet lined with some baking paper. Bake for about 20-25 minutes.

Nutrition information per serving: Kcal: 265, Protein: 1.5g, Carbs: 21g, Fats: 18g

61.   Cherry Parfait

Ingredients:

- 2 tbsp of cherry extract

- 2 cups of milk

- 2 tbsp of low fat cream

- 1 whole egg

- 2 egg whites

- 1 tbsp of honey

- ½ cup of fresh cherries

Preparation:

Gently warm the milk over a minimum heat. Add cream and stir well. You don't want it to boil! Remove from the heat and add cherry extract. Stir until the cream melts. Set side and allow it to cool for a while. Now add egg and egg whites, honey and fresh cherries. Stir well for several minutes and pour into tall glasses. Freeze overnight and serve.

Nutrition information per serving: Kcal: 380, Protein: 4g, Carbs: 58.5g, Fats: 14.5g

62. Frozen Cream with Blueberries

Ingredients:

- 1 cup of low fat cream

- 1 cup of fresh blueberries

- ¼ cup of skim milk

- 2 egg whites

- 1 tbsp of honey

- 1 tsp of brown sugar

Preparation:

Combine the ingredients in a large bowl. Beat well with a fork. Put it in a freezer for about 30 minutes. This creamy mixture is a perfect healthy substitute for ice cream.

Nutrition information per serving: Kcal: 92.5, Protein: 1.5g, Carbs: 17.5g, Fats: 3g

63.   Turkish Sutlac

Ingredients:

- ½ cup of uncooked rice

- 2 cups of milk

- ¼ tsp of salt

- 1 tsp of cinnamon

- ½ tbsp of sugar- free vanilla extract

Preparation:

Use package instructions to cook the rice. In a medium sized saucepan bring 2 cups of milk to boil. Add cooked rice, salt, vanilla extract, and stir well. Cook for about 20 minutes, or until you get a creamy mixture. Stir in some cinnamon and remove from the heat. Allow it to cool in the refrigerator before serving.

Nutrition information per serving: Kcal: 163.5, Protein: 4g, Carbs: 28.5g, Fats: 3.5g

64. Cherry Dessert

Ingredients:

- 2 cup of fresh cherries

- 4 cups of water

- 5 tbsp of brown sugar

- 1 cup of cornstarch

Preparation:

Boil the water and add sugar. Mix well for several minutes and add cherries. Cook for about 15 minutes. Add cornstarch and cook for another 2 minutes. Pour into bowls and allow it to cool.

Nutrition information per serving: Kcal: 80, Protein: 1g, Carbs: 25g, Fats: 1g

65.   Creamy Vanilla with Strawberries

Ingredients:

- 3 large bananas

- 2 cups of skim milk

- ½ cup of water

- 1 tsp of sugar-free vanilla extract

- 1 tsp of cinnamon

- 1 tbsp of cornstarch

- 1 cup of fresh strawberries

- ¼ cup of fresh blueberries

- ½ cup of fat-free whipped dessert topping

Preparation:

Pour the milk into a medium-sized pot. Over a medium-low heat, gently bring it to a boil. Meanwhile peel the banana and mash with a fork. Transfer to a bowl and add vanilla extract and cinnamon. Mix well again and combine with milk. You can add some water if necessary.

Cook for about five minutes, stirring constantly. Now add cornstarch and mix well. Remove from the heat and mix well for a couple of minutes.

Cool for a while and transfer to a fridge. Let it stand for about an hour before serving.

Top with fresh strawberries, blueberries, and whipped dessert topping.

Nutrition information per serving: Kcal: 180, Protein: 6.5g, Carbs: 29g, Fats: 5.5g

66.   Avocado and Cocoa Mousse

Ingredients:

- 1 medium ripe avocado, peeled and pitted
- 4 bananas
- 1 ½ cup of milk
- 1 tsp of vanilla extract
- 1 tbsp of cornstarch
- 1 tbsp of cocoa
- 1 tbsp of brown sugar

Preparation:

Mix the ingredients with food processor. Cool well before serving.

Nutrition information per serving: Kcal: 210, Protein: 2g, Carbs: 31g, Fats: 12g

JUICES

1.   Ginger Carrot Juice

Ingredients:

1 small ginger knob, peeled

1 medium-sized carrot, sliced

1 medium-sized fennel bulb

½ cup of cabbage, torn

Preparation:

Peel the ginger knob and cut into small pieces. Set aside.

Wash and peel the carrot. Cut into thin slices and set aside.

Wash the fennel and trim off the green ends. Using a sharp paring knife, remove the outer layer. Cut into small pieces and set aside. Wash the cabbage thoroughly and torn into small pieces. Set aside. Now, combine ginger, carrot, fennel, and cabbage in a juicer and process until juiced. Transfer to a serving glass and refrigerate before serving.

Nutrition information per serving: Kcal: 72, Protein: 4g, Carbs: 25.9g, Fats: 0.7g

2.   Broccoli Apple Juice

Ingredients:

1 cup of broccoli, chopped

1 small Granny Smith's apple, cored

1 cup of green grapes

1 cup of fresh spinach, torn

1 tbsp fresh mint, finely chopped

Preparation:

Using a large colander, rinse the broccoli and spinach under cold running water. Drain and torn the spinach in small pieces. Trim off the outer leaves of the broccoli and cut into small pieces. Fill the measuring cups and set aside.

Wash the apple and cut lengthwise in half. Remove the core and cut into bite-sized pieces. Set aside. Wash the grapes and remove the stem. Set aside. Now, combine spinach, broccoli, apple, and grapes in a juicer and process until well juiced. Transfer to a serving glass and sprinkle with some fresh mint. Refrigerate for 5 minutes before serving.

Nutrition information per serving: Kcal: 176, Protein: 9.8g, Carbs: 49.5g, Fats:1.7g

3.   Beet Pomegranate Juice

Ingredients:

1 cup of beets, sliced

1 cup of beet greens, chopped

1 cup of pomegranate seeds

1 cup of crookneck squash, sliced

1 cup of celery, chopped

1 tbsp of honey

Preparation:

Wash the beets and trim off the green parts. Cut into bite-sized pieces and set aside.

Use the trimmed beet greens and roughly chop it.

Cut the top of the pomegranate fruit using a sharp knife. Slice down to each of the white membranes inside of the fruit. Pop the seeds into a measuring cup and set aside.

Wash the crookneck squash and cut in half. Scoop out the seeds using a spoon. Cut into small chunks and set aside. Reserve the rest for another juice.

Wash the celery and cut into small pieces. Set aside.

Now, process beets, beet greens, pomegranate seeds, squash, and celery in a juicer.

Transfer to serving glasses and stir in the honey.

Add some ice and serve immediately.

Nutritional information per serving: Kcal: 132, Protein: 6.4g, Carbs: 48.8g, Fats: 1.8g

4.   Carrot Collard Green Juice

Ingredients:

1 large carrot, chopped

1 cup of collard greens, torn

1 cup of avocado, chunked

1 cup of Romaine lettuce, shredded

1 whole cucumber, sliced

¼ tsp of ginger, ground

Preparation:

Wash and peel the carrot. Cut into thin slices and set aside.

Combine collard greens and lettuce in a large colander. Wash thoroughly under cold running water. Drain and shred. Set aside.

Peel the avocado and cut lengthwise in half. Remove the pit and cut into small chunks. Fill the measuring cup and reserve the rest in the refrigerator.

Wash the cucumber and cut into thin slices. Fill the measuring cup and reserve the rest for later. Set aside.

Now, combine carrot, collard greens, avocado, lettuce, and

cucumber in a juicer and process until juiced. Transfer to a serving glass and stir in the ginger.

Refrigerate for 5 minutes before serving.

Nutrition information per serving: Kcal: 271, Protein: 7.3g, Carbs: 34.1g, Fats: 22.8g

5.   Cucumber Orange Juice

Ingredients:

1 cup of cucumber, sliced

1 large orange, peeled and wedged

1 cup of pumpkin, cubed

1 large carrot, sliced

1 small ginger knob, chopped

Preparation:

Wash the cucumber and cut into thin slices. Fill the measuring cup and reserve the rest for later. Set aside.

Peel the orange and divide into wedges. Cut each wedge in half and set aside.

Cut the top of a pumpkin. Cut lengthwise in half and then scrape out the seeds. Cut one large wedge and peel it. Cut into small cubes and fill the measuring cup. Reserve the rest in the refrigerator.

Wash and peel the carrot. Cut into thin slices and set aside.

Peel the ginger knob and cut into small pieces. Set aside.

Now, combine pumpkin, carrot, cucumber, orange, and

ginger in a juicer. Process until well juiced. Transfer to a serving glass and add some ice.

Serve immediately.

Nutrition information per serving: Kcal: 130, Protein: 4.1g, Carbs: 39.1g, Fats: 0.6g

6.   Mango Honey Juice

Ingredients:

1 cup of mango, chunked

1 tbsp of liquid honey

1 whole guava, chopped

1 whole lime, peeled

1 cup of cucumber, sliced

1 medium-sized Golden Delicious apple, cored

Preparation:

Wash and peel the mango. Cut into small chunks and set aside.

Peel the guava using a sharp paring knife. Cut into bite-sized pieces and set aside.

Peel the lime and cut lengthwise in half. Set aside.

Wash the cucumber and cut into thin slices. fill the measuring cup and reserve the rest in the refrigerator.

Wash the apple and cut lengthwise in half. Remove the core and cut into bite-sized pieces. Set aside.

Now, combine mango, guava, lime, cucumber, and apple in a juicer and process until well juiced. Transfer to a serving glass and stir in the honey. Add some crushed ice and serve immediately.

Nutrition information per serving: Kcal: 211, Protein: 3.7g, Carbs: 61.1g, Fats: 1.5g

7.   Lime Banana Juice

Ingredients:

1 whole lime, peeled

1 large banana, sliced

1 cup of blueberries

1 cup of Romaine lettuce, shredded

1 whole cucumber, sliced

Preparation:

Peel the lime and cut lengthwise in half. Set aside.

Peel the banana and cut into thin slices. Set aside.

Rinse the blueberries using a small colander. Slightly drain and fill the measuring cup. Set aside.

Rinse the lettuce thoroughly under cold running water. Shred it and fill the measuring cup. Set aside.

Wash the cucumber and cut into thin slices. Set aside.

Now, combine blueberries, lime, banana, lettuce, and cucumber in a juicer and process until juiced. Transfer to a serving glass and add some crushed ice.

Serve immediately.

Nutrition information per serving: Kcal: 176, Protein: 9.8g, Carbs: 49.5g, Fats: 1.7g

8.   Turnip Beet Juice

Ingredients:

1 cup of turnip greens, torn

1 cup of beets, sliced

5 medium-sized tomatoes, peeled

1 cup of watercress, torn

1 tsp of salt

Preparation:

Wash the beets and trim off the green parts. Cut into small pieces and set aside.

Wash the tomatoes and place them in a bowl. Cut into quarters and reserve the juice while cutting. Set aside.

Combine watercress and turnip greens in a colander and wash under cold running water. Torn with hands and set aside.

Now, combine tomatoes, watercress, turnip greens, and beets in a juicer and process until juiced.

Transfer to serving glasses and stir in the reserved tomato juice, water, and salt.

Refrigerate for 5 minutes before serving.

Nutritional information per serving: Kcal: 212, Protein: 11.7g, Carbs: 62.7g, Fats: 2.2g

9.   Brussels Sprout Lime Juice

Ingredients:

1 cup of Brussels sprouts, halved

1 whole lime, peeled

1 large green bell pepper, chopped

1 cup of broccoli, chopped

2 large carrots, sliced

¼ tsp turmeric, ground

Preparation:

Wash the bell pepper and cut lengthwise in half. Remove the stem and seeds. Chop into small pieces and set aside.

Wash the Brussels sprouts and broccoli. Trim off the wilted and outer leaves. Transfer all to a heavy-bottomed pot and add water enough to cover all. Bring it to a boil and then remove from the heat. Drain well and chop into small pieces. Set aside to cool completely.

Peel the lime and cut lengthwise in half. Set aside.

Wash and peel the carrots. Cut into thin slices and set aside.

Now, combine Brussels sprouts, lime, bell pepper, broccoli, and carrots in a juicer and process until juiced. Transfer to a serving glasses and stir in the turmeric. Add some water, if needed.

Sprinkle with some salt, but it's optional.

Nutrition information per serving: Kcal: 122, Protein: 8.5g, Carbs: 39.1g, Fats: 1.2g

10.   Basil Cucumber Juice

Ingredients:

1 cup of fresh basil, torn

1 cup of cucumber, sliced

1 medium-sized zucchini, chopped

1 cup of red leaf lettuce, torn

1 cup of avocado, cut into bite-sized pieces

Preparation:

Combine basil and lettuce in a large colander and rinse under cold running water. Drain and torn with hands into small pieces. Set aside.

Wash the cucumber and cut into thin slices. Fill the measuring cup and refrigerate for later. Peel the zucchini and chop into small pieces. Set aside. Peel the avocado and cut lengthwise in half. Remove the pit and cut into bite-sized pieces. Fill the measuring cup and reserve the rest in the refrigerator. Now, combine basil, cucumber, lettuce, zucchini, and avocado in a juicer. Process until well juiced. Transfer to a serving glass and add some ice.

Nutrition information per serving: Kcal: 234, Protein: 6.7g, Carbs: 21.7g, Fats: 22.3g

11.   Zucchini Carrot Juice

Ingredients:

1 medium-sized zucchini, sliced

1 large carrot, sliced

1 cup of fresh basil, chopped

1 large yellow bell pepper, chopped

¼ tsp of ginger, ground

Preparation:

Wash the zucchini and cut into small chunks. Set aside.

Wash and peel the carrot. Cut into thin slices and set aside.

Wash the basil thoroughly under cold running water. Slightly drain and chop into small pieces. Set aside. Wash the bell pepper and cut lengthwise in half. Remove the stem and seeds. Cut into small pieces and set aside. Now, combine zucchini, carrot, basil, and pepper in a juicer and process until juiced. Transfer to a serving glass and stir in the ginger. Add some water if needed. Refrigerate for 5 minutes before serving.

Nutrition information per serving: Kcal: 94, Protein: 5.6g, Carbs: 25.4g, Fats: 1.3g

12.   Radish Cucumber Juice

Ingredients:

2 large radishes, chopped

1 cup of cucumber, sliced

1 cup of fresh spinach, torn

1 cup of arugula, torn

¼ tsp turmeric, ground

Preparation:

Wash the radishes and trim off the green parts. Peel and cut into thin slices. Set aside.

Wash the cucumber and cut into thin slices. Set aside.

Wash the spinach thoroughly under cold running water. Slightly drain and torn with hands. Set aside. Wash the arugula and torn with hands. Set aside. Now, combine radish, cucumber, spinach, and arugula in a juicer and process until juiced. Transfer to a serving glass and stir in the turmeric. Refrigerate for 10 minutes before serving.

Nutrition information per serving: Kcal: 53, Protein: 9.4g, Carbs: 15.3g, Fats: 1.1g

13.   Spinach Lemon Juice

Ingredients:

1 cup of spinach, torn

1 whole lemon, peeled

1 cup of strawberries, chopped

1 whole lime, peeled

1 tbsp honey, raw

2 oz of water

Preparation:

Wash the spinach thoroughly under cold running water. Slightly drain and torn into small pieces. Set aside.

Peel the lemon and lime. Cut each fruit lengthwise in half and set aside.

Wash the strawberries and remove the stems. Cut into bite-sized pieces and set aside.

Now, combine spinach, lemon, lime, and strawberries in a juicer and process until juiced. Transfer to a serving glass and stir in the water and honey.

Garnish with some mint, but it's optional.

Refrigerate for 10 minutes before serving.

Enjoy!

Nutrition information per serving: Kcal: 81, Protein: 5.8g, Carbs: 27.8g, Fats: 1.4g

14.   Grapefruit Mint Juice

Ingredients:

1 whole grapefruit

1 cup of fresh mint, torn

1 cup of cantaloupe, cubed

¼ tsp of cinnamon, ground

1 oz coconut water

Preparation:

Peel the grapefruit and divide into wedges. Cut each wedge in half and set aside.

Wash the mint thoroughly and torn with hands into small pieces. Set aside. Cut the cantaloupe in half. Scoop out the seeds and flesh. Cut and peel one large wedge. Chop into chunks and fill the measuring cup. Reserve the rest of the cantaloupe in a refrigerator. Now, combine grapefruit, mint, and cantaloupe in a juicer. Process until well juiced.

Transfer to a serving glass and stir in the cinnamon and coconut water. Add some ice and serve immediately.

Nutrition information per serving: Kcal: 144, Protein: 4.2g, Carbs: 42.6g, Fats: 0.9g

15.   Spinach Cranberry Juice

Ingredients:

1 cup of baby spinach, torn

1 cup of cranberries

1 cup of cantaloupe, diced

1 cup of parsley, chopped

1 medium-sized cucumber, peeled

1 tbsp of honey, raw

Preparation:

Combine spinach and parsley in a colander and wash under cold running water. Torn with hands and set aside.

Wash the cranberries and set aside.

Cut the cantaloupe in half. Scoop out the seeds and flesh. Cut two wedges and peel them. Chop into chunks and set aside. Reserve the rest of the cantaloupe in a refrigerator.

Wash the cucumber and cut into thick slices. Set aside.

Now, process baby spinach, cranberries, cantaloupe, parsley, and cucumber in a juicer.

Transfer to serving glasses and stir in the honey.

Refrigerate for 5 minutes before serving.

Enjoy!

Nutritional information per serving: Kcal: 197, Protein: 10.2g, Carbs: 58.3g, Fats: 2.2g

16.   Apple Banana Juice

Ingredients:

1 medium-sized Granny Smith's apple, cored

1 large banana, chunked

1 cup of pomegranate seeds

1 tbsp of liquid honey

1 oz of water

Preparation:

Wash the apple and cut lengthwise in half. Remove the core and cut into bite-sized pieces. Set aside. Peel the banana and cut into small chunks. Set aside. Cut the top of the pomegranate fruit using a sharp paring knife. Slice down to each of the white membranes inside of the fruit. Pop the seeds into a measuring cup and set aside.

Now, combine apple, banana, and pomegranate seeds in a juicer and process until juiced. Transfer to a serving glass and stir in the honey and water.

Nutrition information per serving: Kcal: 243, Protein: 3.6g, Carbs: 70.1g, Fats: 1.8g

17.   Peach Apple Juice

Ingredients:

1 large peach, pitted and chopped

1 small green apple, cored and chopped

1 cup of banana, sliced

¼ tsp of cinnamon, ground

1 oz of coconut water

1 tbsp of mint, finely chopped

Preparation:

Wash the peach and cut lengthwise in half. Remove the pit and cut into bite-sized pieces. Set side. Wash the apple and cut in half. Remove the core and chop into small pieces. Set aside. Peel the bananas and cut into thin slices. Fill the measuring cup and reserve the rest in the refrigerator. Now, combine peach, apple, and bananas in a juicer and process until well juiced. Transfer to a serving glass and stir in the cinnamon and coconut water. Add some crushed ice and sprinkle with finely chopped mint for some extra taste.

Nutrition information per serving: Kcal: 362, Protein: 5.5g, Carbs: 104g, Fats: 1.7g

18.   Papaya Cabbage Juice

Ingredients:

1 cup of papaya, chopped

1 cup of cabbage, torn

1 cup of red leaf lettuce, torn

2 whole kiwis, peeled

1 whole lime, peeled

1 tsp of coconut sugar

½ cup of pure coconut water, unsweetened

Preparation:

Peel the papaya and cut lengthwise in half. Scoop out the black seeds and flesh using a spoon. Cut into small chunks and set aside.

Combine cabbage and lettuce in a colander and wash under cold running water. Torn with hands and set aside.

Peel the kiwis and lime and cut lengthwise in half. Set aside.

Now, process papaya, cabbage, lettuce, kiwis, and lime in a juicer.

Transfer to serving glasses and coconut water and coconut sugar.

Add some ice and serve immediately.

Nutritional information per serving: Kcal: 201, Protein: 7g, Carbs: 61.7g, Fats: 1.7g

19.   Beet Carrot Juice

Ingredients:

1 cup of beets, trimmed

1 large carrot, sliced

1 cup of avocado, chopped

1 small ginger knob

¼ tsp turmeric, ground

2 oz water

Preparation:

Trim off the green parts of the beets. Slightly peel and cut into thin slices. Fill the measuring cup and refrigerate the rest.

Wash and peel the carrot. Cut into bite-sized pieces and set aside.

Peel the avocado and cut lengthwise in half. Remove the pit and cut into bite-sized pieces. Fill the measuring cup and reserve the rest in the refrigerator.

Peel the ginger knob and cut into small pieces. Set aside.

Now, combine beets, carrot, avocado, and ginger in a

juicer. Process until well juiced and transfer to a serving glass. Stir in the turmeric and water and refrigerate for 10 minutes before serving.

Enjoy!

Nutrition information per serving: Kcal: 265, Protein: 5.9g, Carbs: 33.4g, Fats: 21.8g

20. Cherry Banana Juice

Ingredients:

1 cup of fresh cherries, pitted

1 small banana, peeled

2 cups of green grapes

1 whole lime, peeled

1 tbsp of coconut water

Preparation:

Rinse the cherries using a colander. Drain and cut each in half. Remove the pits and fill the measuring cup. Reserve the rest in the refrigerator.

Peel the banana and cut into chunks. Set aside. Rinse the grapes under cold running water and remove the stems. Set aside. Peel the lime and cut lengthwise in half. Set aside. Now, combine cherries, banana, grapes, and lime in a juicer and process until juiced. Transfer to a serving glass and stir in the coconut water.

Serve immediately.

Nutrition information per serving: Kcal: 292, Protein: 4.1g, Carbs: 82.9g, Fats: 1.3g

21. Cauliflower Celery Juice

Ingredients:

1 cup of cauliflower, chopped

1 cup of celery, chopped

1 cup of asparagus, chopped

1 cup of cucumber, sliced

¼ tsp of turmeric, ground

¼ tsp of cayenne pepper, ground

Preparation:

Wash the cauliflower and trim off the outer leaves. Chop into small pieces and fill the measuring cup. Reserve the rest for later.

Wash the celery and chop into bite-sized pieces. Set aside.

Wash the asparagus under cold running water. Trim off the woody ends and chop into bite-sized pieces. Set aside.

Wash the cucumber and cut into thin slices. Fill the measuring cup and reserve the rest in the refrigerator.

Now, combine cauliflower, celery, asparagus, and cucumber in a juicer and process until juiced. Transfer to a serving glass and stir in the turmeric and cayenne pepper.

Serve immediately.

Nutrition information per serving: Kcal: 52, Protein: 6.1g, Carbs: 15.4g, Fats: 0.7g

22. Zucchini Lemon Juice

Ingredients:

1 medium-sized zucchini, chopped

1 whole lemon, peeled

1 cup of fresh kale, chopped

1 whole lime, peeled

1 cup of fresh mint, torn

Preparation:

Wash the zucchini and cut into small pieces. Set aside.

Peel the lemon and lime. Cut lengthwise in half and set aside.

Rinse the kale thoroughly under cold running water. Drain and chop into small pieces. Set aside. Wash the mint and chop into small pieces. Set aside. Now, combine kale, zucchini, lemon, lime, and mint in a juicer. Process until well juiced. Transfer to a serving glass and add some crushed ice. Serve immediately.

Nutrition information per serving: Kcal: 79, Protein: 7g, Carbs: 24.7g, Fats: 1.7g

23.   Spinach Brussels Sprout Juice

Ingredients:

2 cups of spinach, chopped

1 cup of Brussels sprouts, chopped

1 cup of red bell pepper, chopped

1 large red delicious apple, peeled and cored

¼ tsp of ginger, freshly ground

Preparation:

Wash the spinach thoroughly and torn with hands. Set aside.

Wash the Brussels sprouts and trim off the outer layers. Cut in half and set aside.

Wash the bell pepper and cut lengthwise in half. Remove the seeds and chop into small pieces. Set aside.

Wash the apple and remove the core. Cut into bite-sized pieces and set aside.

Now, combine spinach, Brussels sprouts, bell pepper, and apple in a juicer.

Transfer to serving glasses and stir in the honey.

Add some ice and serve immediately.

Nutritional information per serving: Kcal: 196, Protein: 6.8g, Carbs: 55.6g, Fats: 1.4g

24.   Radish Zucchini Juice

Ingredients:

3 large radishes, chopped

1 small zucchini, sliced

1 cup of avocado, cubed

1 cup of celery, chopped

1 cup of cucumber, sliced

¼ tsp of salt

1 oz of water

Preparation:

Wash the radishes and cut into small pieces. Set aside.

Wash the zucchini and cut into thin slices. Set aside.

Peel the avocado and cut in half. Remove the pit and cut into small cubes. Fill the measuring cup and reserve the rest for later.

Wash the celery and chop it into bite-sized pieces. Set aside.

Wash the cucumber and cut into thin slices. Fill the

measuring cup and reserve the rest for later. Set aside.

Now, combine radishes, zucchini, avocado, celery, and cucumber in a juicer and process until juiced. Transfer to a serving glass and stir in the salt and water.

Serve cold.

Nutrition information per serving: Kcal: 235, Protein: 5.6g, Carbs: 22.3g, Fats: 22.6g

25.   Cantaloupe Apple Juice

Ingredients:

1 large wedge of cantaloupe

1 small green apple, cored

1 cup of pomegranate seeds

1 small ginger knob, sliced

1 oz of water

Preparation:

Cut the cantaloupe in half. Scrape out the seeds and cut one one large wedge. Peel and chop into small pieces. Wrap the rest in a plastic foil and refrigerate for later.

Wash the apple and cut lengthwise in half. Remove the core and cut into bite-sized pieces. Set aside.

Cut the top of the pomegranate fruit using a sharp paring knife. Slice down to each of the white membranes inside of the fruit. Pop the seeds into a measuring cup and set aside.

Peel the ginger and cut into small pieces. Set aside.

Now, combine cantaloupe, apple, pomegranate, and ginger in a juicer. Process until well juiced and transfer to a serving glass. Add some water to adjust the bitterness, if needed.

Refrigerate for 10 minutes before serving.

Nutrition information per serving: Kcal: 162, Protein: 3.1g, Carbs: 45.3g, Fats: 1.5g

26.   Apricot Apple Juice

Ingredients:

3 whole apricots, chopped

1 large green apple, cored

2 whole kiwis, peeled and halved

1 large banana, chunked

Preparation:

Wash the apricots and cut in half. Remove the pits and cut into small pieces. Set aside.

Wash the apple and cut lengthwise in half. Remove the core and cut into bite-sized pieces. Set aside.

Peel the kiwi and cut lengthwise in half. Set aside.

Peel the banana and cut into small chunks. Set aside.

Now, combine apricots, apple, kiwi, and banana in a juicer and process until juiced. Transfer to a serving glass and add some ice.

Serve immediately.

Nutrition information per serving: Kcal: 313, Protein: 5.4g, Carbs: 91g, Fats: 1.9g

27.   Pumpkin Lemon Juice

Ingredients:

1 cup of pumpkin, cubed

1 whole lemon, peeled

1 cup of broccoli, chopped

1 cup of fennel, chopped

1 cup of cucumber, sliced

Preparation:

Cut the top of a pumpkin. Cut lengthwise in half and then scrape out the seeds. Cut one large wedge and peel it. Cut into small cubes and fill the measuring cup. Reserve the rest in the refrigerator.

Peel the lemon and cut lengthwise in half. Set aside.

Wash the broccoli and trim off the outer leaves. Cut into bite-sized pieces and fill the measuring cup. Reserve the rest for later.

Trim off the outer wilted layers of the fennel. Roughly chop it and fill the measuring cup. Reserve the rest for later.

Wash the cucumber and cut into thin slices. Fill the

measuring cup and reserve the rest in the refrigerator. Set aside.

Now, combine pumpkin, lemon, broccoli, fennel, and cucumber in a juicer and process until well juiced. Transfer to a serving glass and add some crushed ice.

Serve immediately.

Nutrition information per serving: Kcal: 196, Protein: 2.8g, Carbs: 55.5g, Fats: 1.3g

28.   Parsley Grapefruit Juice

Ingredients:

2 cups of parsley, chopped

1 whole grapefruit, peeled

1 cup of watermelon, diced

7 oz of green beans, chopped

½ cup of pure coconut water

Preparation:

Wash the parsley under cold running water. Torn with hands and set aside.

Peel the grapefruit and cut into small pieces. Set aside.

Cut the watermelon lengthwise. For one cup, you will need about 1 large wedge. Peel and cut into chunks. Remove the seeds and set aside. Reserve the rest of the melon for some other juices.

Wash the green beans and chop into small pieces. Place them in a pot of boiling water and cook for 3 minutes. Remove from the heat and drain. Set aside.

Now, process, parsley, grapefruit, watermelon, and beans

in a juicer.

Transfer to serving glasses and stir in the coconut water.

Add some ice and serve immediately.

Nutritional information per serving: Kcal: 161, Protein: 6.4g, Carbs: 45.6g, Fats: 1.5g

29. Cauliflower Brussels Sprout Juice

Ingredients:

1 cup of cauliflower, chopped

1 cup of Brussels sprouts, halved

1 large red bell pepper, chopped

¼ tsp of ginger, ground

1 oz of water

Preparation:

Trim off the outer leaves of a cauliflower. Wash it and cut into small pieces. Fill the measuring cup and reserve the rest in the refrigerator. Wash the Brussels sprouts and trim off the wilted layers. Cut each in half and fill the measuring cup. Set aside. Wash the bell pepper and cut lengthwise in half. Remove the seeds and the top stem. Cut into small pieces and set aside. Now, combine cauliflower, Brussels sprouts, and pepper in a juicer and process until juiced. Transfer to a serving glass and stir in the water and ginger.

Serve immediately.

Nutrition information per serving: Kcal: 106, Protein: 9.6g, Carbs: 30.9g, Fats: 1.3g

30.   Pear Plum Juice

Ingredients:

1 large pear, cored

1 whole plum, pitted and chopped

1 cup of raspberries

1 medium-sized Granny Smith's apple, cored

¼ tsp of cinnamon, ground

1 oz of coconut water

Preparation:

Wash the pear and cut lengthwise in half. Remove the core and cut into small pieces. Set aside.

Wash the plum and cut in half. Remove the pit and set aside.

Wash the raspberries using a small colander. Slightly drain and set aside.

Wash the apple and cut in half. Remove the core and cut into bite-sized pieces. Set aside.

Now, combine pear, plum, raspberries, and apple in a juicer and process until well juiced. Transfer to a serving glass and stir in the cinnamon and coconut water. Add some crushed ice and serve immediately.

Enjoy!

Nutrition information per serving: Kcal: 239, Protein: 3.5g, Carbs: 79.9g, Fats: 1.6g

31. Mint Apple Juice

Ingredients:

1 cup of fresh mint, torn

1 small Red Delicious apple, cored

1 cup of mango, chunked

1 medium-sized peach, pitted

Preparation:

Wash the mint thoroughly under cold running water and torn with hands. Set aside. You can soak mint in hot water for 2 minutes, but it's optional.

Wash the apple and cut lengthwise in half. Remove the core and cut into bite-sized pieces. Set aside. Peel the mango and cut into small chunks. Fill the measuring cup and reserve the rest in the refrigerator. Wash the peach and cut in half. Remove the pit and cut into small pieces. Set aside. Now, combine mint, apple, mango, and peach in a juicer and process until well juiced. Transfer to a serving glass and add few ice cubes.

Serve immediately.

Nutrition information per serving: Kcal: 227, Protein: 4.1g, Carbs: 64.9g, Fats: 1.6g

32.   Banana Apple Juice

Ingredients:

1 large banana, peeled and chunked

1 small Granny Smith's apple, cored

1 cup of fresh kale, chopped

1 cup of Brussels sprouts, halved

¼ tsp of ginger, ground

1 oz of coconut water

Preparation:

Peel the banana and cut into small chunks. Set aside.

Wash the apple and cut in half. Remove the core and cut into bite-sized pieces. Set aside.

Wash the kale thoroughly under cold running water and slightly drain. Chop into small pieces and set aside.

Wash the Brussels sprouts and remove the outer wilted layers. Cut each in half and set aside.

Now, combine banana, apple, kale, and Brussels sprouts in a juicer and process until juiced. Transfer to a serving glass and stir in the coconut water and ginger.

Add some ice and serve immediately.

Nutrition information per serving: Kcal: 223, Protein: 7.9g, Carbs: 64.4g, Fats: 1.6g

33. Lemon Artichoke Juice

Ingredients:

1 whole lemon, peeled

1 medium-sized artichoke, chopped

1 cup of fresh cherries, pitted

1 medium-sized apple, cored

¼ tsp of cinnamon, ground

Preparation:

Peel the lemon and cut lengthwise in half. Set aside.

Wash the artichoke and trim off the outer, hard leaves. Cut into bite-sized pieces and set aside. Wash the cherries using a large colander. Cut each in half and remove the pits. Set aside. Wash the apple and cut lengthwise in half. Remove the core and cut into bite-sized pieces. Set aside.

Now, combine lemon, artichoke, cherries, and apple in a juicer and process until juiced. Transfer to a serving glass and stir in the cinnamon.

Refrigerate for 5 minutes before serving.

Nutrition information per serving: Kcal: 205, Protein: 7.2g, Carbs: 66.2g, Fats: 0.9g

34.   Apricot Turmeric Juice

Ingredients:

2 whole apricots, pitted

¼ tsp of turmeric, ground

2 whole grapefruits

1 cup of collard greens, chopped

Preparation:

Wash the apricots and cut lengthwise in half. Remove the pit and cut into bite-sized pieces. Set aside.

Peel the grapefruits and divide into wedges. Cut each wedge in half and set aside. Wash the collard greens thoroughly under cold running water. Drain and chop into small pieces. Set aside. Now, combine apricots, grapefruit, and collard greens in a juicer and process until juiced. Transfer to a serving glass and stir in the turmeric.

Refrigerate for 5 minutes before serving.

Nutrition information per serving: Kcal: 208, Protein: 5.8g, Carbs: 62.1g, Fats: 1.2g

35.   Raspberry Lemon Juice

Ingredients:

1 cup of raspberries

1 whole lemon, peeled

1 cup of beets, sliced

1 medium-sized pear, chopped

1 oz of water

Preparation:

Rinse well the raspberries using a small colander. Drain and set aside.

Peel the lemon and cut lengthwise in half. Set aside.

Wash the beets and trim off the green parts. Cut into thin slices and fill the measuring cup. Reserve the rest for later. Wash the pear and cut in half. Remove the core and cut into bite-sized pieces. Set aside. Now, combine raspberries, lemon, beets, and pear in a juicer and process until juiced. Transfer to a serving glass and stir in the water.

Refrigerate for 5 minutes before serving.

Nutrition information per serving: Kcal: 165, Protein: 4.9g, Carbs: 60.2g, Fats: 1.4g

36.   Cucumber Cranberry Juice

Ingredients:

1 cup of cucumber, sliced

1 cup of whole cranberries

1 large wedge of honeydew melon

2 large strawberries

1 oz coconut water

Preparation:

Wash the cucumber and cut into thin slices. Fill the measuring cup and reserve the rest for later. Set aside.

Using a small colander, rinse well the cranberries. Drain and set aside.

Cut melon lengthwise in half. Scoop out the seeds and then wash the melon. Cut one wedge and peel it. Cut into bite-sized pieces and set aside.

Wash the strawberries and remove the stems. Chop into small pieces and set aside.

Now, combine cucumber, cranberries, melon, and strawberries in a juicer. Process until well juiced. Transfer to a serving glass and add few ice cubes.

Serve immediately.

Nutrition information per serving: Kcal: 96, Protein: 1.8g, Carbs: 31.4g, Fats: 0.6g

37.   Spinach Carrot Juice

Ingredients:

1 medium whole tomato, chopped

1 cup of fresh spinach, torn

1 medium-sized carrot, sliced

1 cup of celery, chopped

¼ tsp of salt

¼ tsp of balsamic vinegar

Preparation:

Wash the spinach thoroughly under cold running water. Torn into small pieces and set aside. Wash and peel the carrot. Cut into thin slices and set aside. Wash the tomato and place in a small bowl. Cut into bite-sized pieces. Make sure to reserve the tomato juice while cutting. Set aside. Wash the celery and chop into small pieces. Set aside. Now, combine spinach, carrot, tomato, and celery in a juicer and process until juiced. Transfer to a serving glass and stir in the salt, vinegar, and reserved tomato juice.

Nutrition information per serving: Kcal: 72, Protein: 8.4g, Carbs: 21.2g, Fats: 1.4g

38.   Banana Blackberry Juice

Ingredients:

1 cup of pineapple chunks

1 large banana, sliced

1 cup of blackberries

1 whole lime, peeled

1 oz of water

Preparation:

Peel the banana and cut into thin slices. Set aside.

Place the blackberries in a small colander and wash under cold running water. Slightly drain and set aside. Using a sharp paring knife, cut the top of the pineapple. Gently remove all hard skin and slice it into thin slices. Fill the measuring cup and reserve the rest for later. Peel the lime and cut lengthwise in half. Set aside.

Now, combine banana, blackberries, pineapple, and lime in a juicer. Process until well juiced. Transfer to a serving glass and add some ice before serving.

Nutrition information per serving: Kcal: 222, Protein: 4.5g, Carbs: 70.2g, Fats: 1.4g

39. Lime Apple Juice

Ingredients:

1 whole lime, peeled

1 small Granny Smith's apple, cored

1 cup of strawberries, chopped

1 whole lemon, peeled

2 oz coconut water

¼ tsp cinnamon, ground

Preparation:

Peel the lime and lemon. Cut each fruit in half and set aside.

Wash the apple and cut lengthwise in half. Remove the core and cut into small pieces. Set aside. Wash the strawberries and remove the stems. Cut into bite-sized pieces and fill the measuring cup. Reserve the rest for later. Now, combine lime, lemon, strawberries, and apple in a juicer and process until juiced. Transfer to a serving glass and stir in the coconut water and cinnamon. Add some crushed ice and serve immediately.

Nutrition information per serving: Kcal: 122, Protein: 2.4g, Carbs: 39.7g, Fats: 0.9g

40.   Tomato Watercress Juice

Ingredients:

1 medium whole tomato, chopped

1 cup of watercress, torn

1 large red bell pepper, chopped

1 rosemary sprig

1 oz of water

Preparation:

Wash the tomato and place in a small bowl. Chop into small pieces and make sure to reserve the tomato juice while cutting. Set aside. Wash the watercress thoroughly under cold running water. Slightly drain and torn with hands into small pieces. Set aside. Wash the bell pepper and cut lengthwise in half. Remove the seeds and chop into small pieces. Set aside. Now, combine tomato, watercress, and bell pepper in a juicer and process until juiced. Transfer to a serving glass and stir in the water and reserved tomato juice. Sprinkle with rosemary and serve immediately.

Nutrition information per serving: Kcal: 56, Protein: 3.5g, Carbs: 15.1g, Fats: 0.7g

41.   Celery Lemon Juice

Ingredients:

1 cup of celery, chopped

1 whole lemon, peeled

1 large carrot, sliced

1 small Golden Delicious apple, cored

¼ tsp turmeric, ground

¼ tsp ginger, ground

Preparation:

Wash the celery and cut into small pieces. Set aside.

Peel the lemon and cut lengthwise in half. Set aside.

Wash and peel the carrot. Cut into small slices and set aside. Wash the apple and cut in half. Remove the core and cut into bite-sized pieces. Set aside. Now, combine celery, lemon, carrot, and apple in a juicer and process until juiced. Transfer to a serving glass and stir in the water, turmeric, and ginger. If you like, add some crushed ice.

Nutrition information per serving: Kcal: 105, Protein: 2.4g, Carbs: 32.8g, Fats: 0.7g

42.   Peach Apple Juice

Ingredients:

1 large peach, pitted and chopped

1 medium-sized green apple, cored and chopped

1 cup of watermelon, cubed

1 small banana, chunked

¼ tsp of cinnamon, ground

Preparation:

Wash the peach and cut lengthwise in half. Remove the pit and chop into bite-sized pieces. Set aside.

Wash the apple and cut in half. Remove the core and cut into bite-sized pieces. Set aside.

Cut the watermelon in half. Cut one large wedge and wrap the rest in a plastic foil and refrigerate. Peel the slice and cut into small cubes. Remove the pits and fill the measuring cup. Set aside.

Peel the banana and cut into small chunks. Set aside.

Now, combine watermelon, peach, apple, and banana in a juicer and process until juiced. Transfer to a serving glass and stir in the cinnamon.

Add some ice and serve immediately!

Nutrition information per serving: Kcal: 260, Protein: 4.4g, Carbs: 73.9g, Fats: 1.3g

43.   Cucumber Kale Juice

Ingredients:

1 cup of cucumber, sliced

1 cup of fresh kale, chopped

1 cup of fresh spinach, chopped

1 cup of Swiss chard, torn

¼ tspof ginger, ground

1 oz of water

Preparation:

Wash the cucumber and cut into thin slices. Fill the measuring cup and reserve the rest in the refrigerator. Combine spinach, kale, and Swiss chard in a large colander. Rinse under cold running water and slightly drain. Chop all into small pieces and set aside. Now, combine cucumber, kale, spinach, Swiss chard, in a juicer and process until well juiced. Transfer to a serving glass and stir in the ginger and water. Refrigerate for 5 minutes before serving.

Nutrition information per serving: Kcal: 63, Protein: 9.9g, Carbs: 16.7g, Fats: 1.6g

44.   Strawberry Banana Juice

Ingredients:

1 cup of strawberries, chopped

1 cup of banana, chunked

1 cup of cantaloupe, chopped

2 whole plums, chopped

¼ tsp of cinnamon, ground

Preparation:

Wash the strawberries and remove the stems. Cut into bite-sized pieces and set aside.

Peel the banana and cut into chunks. Fill the measuring cup and reserve the rest. Set aside.

Cut the cantaloupe in half. Scrape out the seeds and cut one one large wedge. Peel and chop into small pieces and fill the measuring cup. Wrap the rest in a plastic foil and refrigerate for later.

Wash the plums and cut each in half. Remove the pits and cut into small pieces. Set aside.

Now, combine strawberries, banana, cantaloupe, and

plums in a juicer and process until juiced. Transfer to a serving glass and stir in the cinnamon.

Add some crushed ice and serve immediately.

Nutrition information per serving: Kcal: 249, Protein: 4.8g, Carbs: 73.1g, Fats: 1.5g

45.   Cabbage Beet Juice

Ingredients:

1 cup of purple cabbage, chopped

1 cup of beets, sliced

1 large red bell pepper, chopped

1 cup of fresh spinach, torn

3 cherry tomatoes, halved

¼ tsp of salt

Preparation:

Combine cabbage and spinach in a large colander. Rinse thoroughly under cold running water and drain. Torn into small pieces and set aside.

Wash the beets and trim off the green parts. Peel and cut into thin slices and fill the measuring cup. Reserve the rest for later.

Wash the bell pepper and cut lengthwise in half. Remove the stem and seeds. Cut into small pieces and set aside.

Wash the cherry tomatoes and remove the stems. Cut into halves and set aside.

Now, combine cabbage, beets, bell pepper, spinach, and tomatoes in a juicer and process until juiced. Transfer to a serving glass and stir in the salt.

Serve immediately.

Nutrition information per serving: Kcal: 134, Protein: 11.5g, Carbs: 39.1g, Fats: 1.8g

46.   Beet Apple Juice

Ingredients:

1 whole beet, chopped

1 small Granny Smith's apple, cored

1 cup of watermelon, cubed

1 tsp lemon extract

Preparation:

Wash and trim off the beet. Cut into bite-sized pieces and set aside.

Wash the apple and cut in half. Remove the core and cut into small pieces. Set aside. Cut the top of the watermelon. Cut lengthwise in half and then cut one large wedge. Peel it and cut into small cubes. Remove the seeds and fill the measuring cup. Wrap the rest in a plastic foil and refrigerate for later. Now, combine beet, apple, and watermelon in a juicer and process until well juiced. Transfer to a serving glass and stir in the lemon extract.

Refrigerate for 10 minutes before serving. Garnish with mint and enjoy!

Nutrition information per serving: Kcal: 138, Protein: 2.8g, Carbs: 38.9g, Fats: 0.6g

ADDITIONAL TITLES FROM THIS AUTHOR

70 Effective Meal Recipes to Prevent and Solve Being Overweight: Burn Fat Fast by Using Proper Dieting and Smart Nutrition

By

Joe Correa CSN

48 Acne Solving Meal Recipes: The Fast and Natural Path to Fixing Your Acne Problems in Less Than 10 Days!

By

Joe Correa CSN

41 Alzheimer's Preventing Meal Recipes: Reduce or Eliminate Your Alzheimer's Condition in 30 Days or Less!

By

Joe Correa CSN

70 Effective Breast Cancer Meal Recipes: Prevent and Fight Breast Cancer with Smart Nutrition and Powerful Foods

By

Joe Correa CSN

www.ingramcontent.com/pod-product-compliance
Lightning Source LLC
Chambersburg PA
CBHW030246030426
42336CB00009B/273